Leadership and management in Healthcare

Leadership and Management in Healthcare

Neil Gopee and Jo Galloway

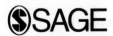

Los Angeles • London • New Delhi • Singapore • Washington DC

SAGE Publications Ltd
1 Oliver's Yard
55 City Road
London EC1Y 1SP

SAGE Publications Inc.
2455 Teller Road
Thousand Oaks, California 91320

SAGE Publications India Pvt Ltd
B 1/I 1 Mohan Cooperative Industrial Area
Mathura Road
New Delhi 110 044

SAGE Publications Asia-Pacific Pte Ltd
33 Pekin Street #02-01
Far East Square
Singapore 048763

Library of Congress Control Number: 2008925096

British Library Cataloguing in Publication data

A catalogue record for this book is available from the British Library

ISBN 978–1–4129–3017–8
ISBN 978–1–4129–3018–5 (pbk)

Typeset by Newgen Imaging Systems (P) Ltd, Chennai, India
Printed in Great Britain by The Cromwell Press Ltd,
Trowbridge, Wiltshire
Printed on paper from sustainable resources

Contents

List of illustrations

Boxes

Figures

Tables

Acknowledgements

With special thanks to Roberto, Robyn, Sacha and Eileen for their ongoing support and encouragement

– Jo Galloway

I extend special thanks to my daughters Hema, Sheila and Neeta for their continuing support with this venture

– Neil Gopee

List of abbreviations

ACL	Action centred leadership
AHP	Allied health professional
CPD	Continuing professional development
CLP	Clinical Leadership Programme
CNO	Chief Nursing Officer
CSW	Clinical support worker (is also referred to as healthcare assistant or healthcare support worker)
DCM	Duty clinical manager
DH	Department of Health
EBHC	Evidence-based healthcare
EPP	Expert patient programme
ICU	Intensive Care Unit
ICP	Integrated care pathways
IDPR	Individual Development and Performance Review (also known as appraisal)
IHI	Institute of Health Improvement
IIP	Investors in People
ITU	Intensive Therapy Unit
IWL	Improving Working Lives
LEO	Leadership Empowered Organisations
MDT	Multi-disciplinary team
MEWS	Modified early warning score
MPE	Manpower equivalent
MBO	Management by objectives
NHS	National Health Service
NHS III	NHS Institute for Innovation and Improvement
NHS KSF	The NHS Knowledge and Skills Framework
NICE	National Institute for Health and Clinical Excellence
NMC	Nursing and Midwifery Council
NSF	National Service Framework
PALS	Patient Advice and Liaison Service
PCT	Primary Care Trust
PREP	Post-registration education and practice
RCT	Randomised controlled trials
RN	Registered Nurse
SAP	Single Assessment Process
SHA	Strategic Health Authority
SWOT	Strengths, weaknesses, opportunities and threats
WTE	Whole time equivalent

Introduction

The months leading up to and after the point of registration can be both an exciting and challenging time for healthcare professionals. Completing final assignments and practice competencies, applying for and securing your first post as a qualified healthcare professional, coping with the accountability and responsibility of your new role as a registered practitioner, ensuring that you get the right support and fit into your new team are to name but a few. This text book has been designed to support you on your journey from an emerging healthcare professional through to becoming a clinical manager.

Leadership and management are essential skills for all qualified healthcare professionals, regardless of the position that they hold. These skills have relevance for everyday practice in delivering care today, and also in leading and managing change and new ways of working for the care that is delivered tomorrow. It is well recognised that if you do what you always do then the results will be the same, however, to effect change we need to work differently. This book has been developed as a composite resource on leadership and management to support the everyday practice of healthcare professionals working at Bands 5 and 6, or their equivalent. It is also intended as an essential resource for emerging practitioners; namely healthcare students who are in the final year of their pre-registration preparation.

From our experience of teaching leadership and management within higher education, we are aware that the majority of books on this subject area within healthcare are either aimed at Ward Manager/Band 7 level, or are based around the healthcare systems of other countries. We recognised the need to have a core text that is set in the context of healthcare that is delivered in the United Kingdom and that also focuses on supporting leadership and management development for new and emerging healthcare professionals. This book is therefore firmly rooted within health care delivery and professional practice within the United Kingdom.

Whilst management and leadership theories are generic and can be applied across disciplines and geographical boundaries, this book will also be of interest to healthcare professionals from other countries, in order to facilitate comparative analysis with the healthcare systems and care delivery within their respective countries.

We recognise that a gap can sometimes exist between what is taught at university and the care that is actually delivered in the practice setting. As authors, we have a strong background of working within clinical practice, managing healthcare and also teaching in Higher Education Institutions. The book has been written with the intention of bridging this theory–practice gap, through drawing upon relevant theories and supporting the reader through action points to apply them to their individual practice settings.

Our shared philosophy is that learning should be enjoyable and that we can all learn something from our everyday experiences and interactions. The book utilises reflection within the action points as a way of supporting you to turn your experiences into learning opportunities. We hope that you find the book to be an invaluable resource to support you in your everyday practice to deliver high quality, person-centred care and to achieve your aspirations.

Organisation of the book

Chapter 1

How does government policy relate to the care that is delivered within my practice setting?

Chapter 1 sets the context for healthcare delivery and will help you to translate this to your practice setting. This chapter will also support you to organise care delivery and ensure effective communication with your patients and colleagues.

Chapter 2

There are so many management theories, how do they relate to me and how can I use them to develop my management skills?

Chapter 2 begins by identifying the everyday management activities of the Duty Clinical Manager (DCM). This chapter will enable you to explore the qualities and personal skills of effective managers and to utilise management theories, roles and styles to best advantage.

Chapter 3

What is the difference between leadership and management and how can I be a good leader?

Effective clinical leadership is essential for the development of healthcare practice and the modernisation of services. This chapter distinguishes management from leadership and provides you with the opportunity to reflect on your practice and support personal leadership development.

Chapter 4

Problem-solving, decision-making and managing conflict, what tools can I draw upon to support my practice?

Healthcare practitioners are faced with a range of decisions that they have to make on a day-to-day basis. This chapter presents you with frameworks for decision-making and problem-solving within the context of professional practice.

Chapter 5

How can quality be improved without providing more time and increasing resources?

Quality improvement is everybody's business and the DCM has a key role in supporting ongoing quality improvement and monitoring. This chapter examines quality frameworks and tools that you can utilise to maximise use of time and improve the quality of care that is delivered within your practice setting.

Chapter 6

Change, change and more change – how can I inspire change and facilitate the change management process at my level in the practice setting?

Change is omnipresent in healthcare and is essential to the modernisation of healthcare services, together with the quest for ongoing improvements to quality and patient outcomes. This chapter critically examines change management theories and provides a framework for you to plan, implement and evaluate change in your practice setting.

Chapter 7

How can I deliver high quality care while ensuring best value for money and working within a set budget?

Healthcare resources need to be effectively and efficiently managed in order to maximise outcomes for patients and ensure best value for money. This chapter addresses both the management of human and consumable resources and supports you to develop budget management skills and a command of financial terminology.

Chapter 8

So many competing priorities, targets to meet and demands on my time – what can I do to ensure that myself and my team members feel supported?

Healthcare professionals have a number of challenges, competing priorities and demands to manage throughout the course of their day-to-day practice. This chapter will support you to identify self-management strategies, support and coping mechanisms to ensure your survival.

Chapter 9

How can I involve patients in their care and work with my team to deliver care that is person-centred?

Current national policy priorities include the provision of personalised care and patient and public involvement in the delivery of healthcare services. This chapter explores the power base of both healthcare professionals and patients, and provides you with opportunities to explore mechanisms to promote patient involvement within the care that is delivered in your practice setting.

Chapter 10

Healthcare is delivered in the context of teams with a shared purpose, how can I be both a good team player and an effective team leader?

Achieving seamless services and ensuring timely transfers of patient care are reliant upon effective team work between primary, secondary, community and social care. This chapter explores team roles and supports you to identify and apply mechanisms to maximise and evaluate team performance.

Chapter 11

How can I teach and support colleagues and healthcare students and also develop my role as an effective leader and manager?

Education, training and personal and professional development are essential to support service development, and ongoing improvements to the quality of care and patient outcomes. The DCM has responsibility for their own development and also to support their colleagues and healthcare students. This chapter will support you to identify development needs and to capitalise on the opportunities that are available.

How to use the book

The book includes a number of features that have been integrated to support your learning and development. These features will support you to utilise the book as a resource that you can come back to again and again to further expand and reinforce your learning.

Action points – Action points are included throughout all of the chapters to support you to reflect on current practice and to learn from your experiences. Action points enable you to apply your learning to practice situations and to look at suggested supporting materials in more depth to enhance the scope of your knowledge in the identified area.

Best practice guidelines – Best practice guidelines are provided at the end of each chapter to highlight the key messages that have been constituted, to inform your practice and for you to apply within your practice setting.

Glossary – A glossary of terms have been incorporated to help you navigate your way around the book and to explore areas of interest in more detail and within different contexts.

Summaries – Summaries are provided at the end of each chapter as an aide memoir and to support you to relocate and revisit pertinent points as required.

Terminology

The following terminology is used throughout the book:

The term **'patient'** is used as a generic term to refer to 'users' of health and social care in the widest sense and therefore also represents service users and clients.

'Practice setting' relates to the locations where healthcare practitioners deliver care, to include wards, clinics, GP surgeries and the patient's own home.

'Care' is used as a generic term that also represents therapy and treatment.

The terms **'healthcare practitioner'**, **'healthcare professional'** and **'registrant'** are used interchangeably to refer to qualified nurses, allied health professionals and health scientists, who are registered with their respective professional body.

'Duty Clinical Manager' is the term used throughout the book to refer to a healthcare professional who has management responsibility for a group of patients, a team of staff, or a practice setting. This responsibility may be for the duration of a span of duty, for example, managing the practice setting, or may be more permanent in nature, for example, managing a team of staff or a group of patients. The term is used as a way of differentiating between the role and responsibilities of the identified figurehead or appointed manager of the practice setting.

ONE Organising daily care within the current context of healthcare provision

Introduction

The roles and functions that healthcare practitioners fulfil can be grouped under five key categories, namely hands-on clinical practice, the management of care, leadership, teaching and utilising research. This chapter focuses on the management component with the aim of ensuring safe and effective care for patients. Ways of organising care are explored, together with the duty clinical manager's (DCM) role in operationalising the various approaches.

The DCM needs to conduct their activities with full consideration of the context and ethos of working in contemporary healthcare. This entails taking full account of government strategy as outlined in, for example, *High Quality Care For All – NHS Next Stage Review Final Report* (Department of Health [DH], 2008a) which builds upon the reforms that have been achieved over the previous decade, and focuses on the achievement of high quality care in all aspects.

Chapter objectives

On completion of this chapter you will be able to:

- enunciate the prevailing social and political contexts in which care and treatment are delivered;
- identify specific healthcare activities that the DCM undertakes over the course of their managerial duties in the practice setting;
- assess the strengths and weaknesses of the various modes of care organisation, and reflect on their relevance to the practice setting; and
- discuss the role of effective communication in care delivery and identify strategies to maximise communication within the practice setting.

The prevailing social and policy context of healthcare provision

Healthcare professions are influenced by major paradigm shifts that currently see healthcare being influenced by DH White Papers, National Service Frameworks (NSF), new government policies, consumer surveys and research. Demographic changes such as an ageing population, the increasing number of people with long-term conditions and rising consumer expectations and demands all need to be addressed.

Government devolution and the creation of national assemblies for Wales and Northern Ireland, together with the Scottish Parliament have had an impact on widening differences in health and social care policy between the four nations. Although policy aims demonstrate similarities across the United Kingdom, each nation has developed its own policy direction to meet the needs of the population it serves.

Current national priorities for healthcare include 'care closer to home', together with a paradigm shift from a more curative focus towards promoting wellness and preventing ill-health. Influential government policy publications in particular have a major impact on the management of care, some of the more significant ones of which are as follows:

- *High Quality Care For All – NHS Next Stage Review Final Report* (DH, 2008a) – builds upon the NHS reforms that have been achieved over the previous decade, and focuses on the achievement of high quality care that is fair, personalised, effective and safe.
- *Our Health, Our Care, Our Say: A New Direction for Community Services* (DH, 2006a) – sets out the Department of Health's vision for the provision of good quality social care and NHS services in the communities where people live. It is part of the government's plan for services to become more responsive to patients' needs and prevent ill health through the promotion of healthy lifestyles. This involves working together with social care services to give people more independence, choice and control.
- *Standards for Better Health* (DH, 2006b) – Initially published in 2004 (updated in 2006), this document signals a move to address the government's national targets and divert focus to standards and to meeting local health priorities.
- *The NHS Knowledge and Skills Framework and the Development Review Process (NHS KSF)* (DH, 2004a) – a framework of job definitions for healthcare employees (except doctors and dentists and some board level and other senior managers).
- *The Wanless Report – Securing Our Future Health: Taking a Long-Term View* (HM Treasury, 2002) – is the first ever independent review and evidence-based assessment of the long-term resource requirements for the NHS.
- *The NHS Plan – A Plan for Investment, a Plan for Reform* (DH, 2000a) – set out the Labour Government's first longer term strategy for the NHS with emphasis on the 'modernisation' of various components of the health service.

The NHS Plan (DH, 2000a) was published three years after the Labour Party returned to power and set out their vision for the NHS in *The New NHS – Modern, Dependable* (DH, 1997). *The NHS Plan* comprises the government's strategic plans for healthcare provision, and therefore the strategic directions the NHS would take on a range of services to be established in subsequent years. It enunciated the nature of a modernised NHS on the basis of ten NHS 'core principles' that were identified to 'reshape the NHS from the patient's point of view' (p. 3). *The NHS Plan* aimed to rectify underfunding in the NHS through increased investment for new hospitals and primary care centres, and an increased number of staff who would be empowered to undertake a wider range of clinical tasks such as running clinics and prescribing drugs.

A progress report was issued four years after the publication of *The NHS Plan*, as *The NHS Improvement Plan: Putting People at the Heart of Public Services* (DH, 2004b), which concluded that *The NHS Plan* was transforming the NHS, with dramatic improvements in key areas in tackling health problems such as cancer and coronary heart disease, and also a reduction in mortality rates. *Standards for Better Health* (DH, 2006b) provides a further update on *The NHS Plan* but with less focus on targets, and more on standards and local healthcare needs.

Various *National Service Frameworks* (NSF) have been developed as 'strategies for improving specific areas of care, which contain measurable goals within set time frames' (DH, 2005a:1), and others are in the process of development. These provide quality assurance tools, with published NSFs in a number of key areas that include coronary heart disease, cancer, mental health, older people, diabetes and long-term conditions. National clinical guidelines and protocols, such as those published by NICE, also support the delivery of high standards of care.

With *Our Health, Our Care, Our Say: A New Direction for Community Services* (DH, 2006a) the aim is to provide good quality social care and NHS services within the communities where patients live, and thus to become more responsive to their healthcare needs and prevent ill health. It comprises key themes that ensued from extensive public consultation, such as putting people more in control of their own health and care, enabling and supporting health, independence and well-being, and rapid and convenient access to high-quality, cost-effective care.

Shaping Healthcare for the Next Decade (DH, 2007a) was initiated on the appointment of the new Prime Minister and Health Secretary in July 2007. Its remit was to carry out a wide-ranging review of the NHS for a well-resourced NHS that is clinically led, patient-centred and locally accountable. This incorporates a change of direction with a plurality of services within inter-professional care, recognition and utilisation of the independent sector as a provider of care, and a resultant widening of patient choice.

High Quality Care for all: NHS Next Stage Final Review (2008a) was published on the 60th Birthday of the NHS and focuses on quality, personalisation and choice within health services. The DCM needs to be able to identify the impact of government health and social care policy for their respective professional disciplines and to translate this within the practice setting in which they work. The government benefits from a number of professional officers who are leaders in their professions and act in an advisory capacity to Department of Health ministers, other government departments and the Prime Minister. Within the Department of Health the professional officers include the Chief Medical Officer, Chief Nursing Officer, Chief Dental Officer, Chief Health Professions Officer, Chief Pharmaceutical Officer and Chief Scientific Officer. All the chief professional officers have their own pages on the Department of Health website where their respective strategies, publications and newsletters can be found.

England's Chief Nursing Officer (CNO), for example, has published a number of key documents pertaining to midwifery and the four branches of nursing. Publications include the *Essence of Care* (DH, 2003) which focuses on improving the essentials of care through benchmarking, and *Modernising Nursing Careers – Setting the Direction* (DH, 2006c), which is the outcome of the work of the four UK Chief Nursing Officers, and addresses the careers of registered nurses (RNs). Other publications are more specific to a branch of nursing or a particular patient group such as *Good Practice in Learning Disability Nursing* (DH, 2007b) which provides good practice guidance to support learning disability nursing to make a major contribution to the health and well-being of people with a learning disability, and *From Values to Action: The Chief Nursing Officer's Review of Mental Health Nursing* (DH, 2006d) which sets out recommendations for shaping the development of mental health nursing, with a focus on improving the outcomes and experience of care for service users and carers.

The healthcare workforce in the twenty-first century

The NHS workforce has been changing for some time in the broader context of employment and changes in society. This includes:

- increasing specialisation and advancing practice;
- an increase in the number of Clinical Support Workers (CSW) as part of workforce redesign;
- changes in shift patterns such as 12-hour shifts; and
- moves in educational preparation leading towards healthcare professions becoming all graduate professions.

Maslin-Prothero (1997:432) explored the prevailing literature on healthcare employment in organisations, and concluded that largely the 'concept of job for life no longer exists'. This is because organisations want an adaptable workforce of individuals who are prepared to be lifelong learners, and who adapt and change as required by the organisation. Various changes that impact on healthcare delivery, including technological, demographic and social attitude changes, are identified in Chapter 6 where the management of change is examined. The development of a variety of transferable skills including skills in critical thinking, problem-solving and reflective practice is seen as essential.

The DCM needs to be aware of the dynamics of employment, whilst ensuring that there are appropriate numbers of staff with appropriate knowledge and skills for care delivery. New roles are also being developed, such as physician's assistant and anaesthetic practitioners which further expand the professional groups that constitute the multi-disciplinary team. Staffing is discussed further in the context of human resource management in Chapter 7, and teamwork in Chapter 10. Furthermore, there are other DH agendas that are at different stages of development that the DCM needs to be cognisant of. These include various policy documents that are to follow the review of the NHS by Lord Darzi (DH, 2008a), and the *Trust, Assurance and Safety – The Regulation of Health Professionals in the 21st Century* (DH, 2007c) that refers to more central regulation of all healthcare professions.

The healthcare practitioner as a DCM

In the light of the healthcare provision contexts just discussed, the DCM's responsibility is firmly grounded in the organisation and management of the care of patients. It is pertinent, however, to determine the various roles of healthcare practitioners within healthcare organisations.

Action point 1.1 – Roles of the DCM, and organising care

Make a list, from your experience, of all the professional activities that a DCM engages in during a span of duty.

You should have been able to identify several professional activities that healthcare practitioners engage in during a span of duty. These may include:

- Managing resources
- Ensuring the health and safety of staff/patients/visitors
- Drug administration
- Hands-on clinical care
- Organising transfers of patient care
- Training and education
- Preceptoring and mentoring
- Participation in risk management initiatives
- Care planning and documentation
- Ensuring evidence-based care
- Care co-ordination/communication with multi-disciplinary team (MDT) members
- Complaints handling
- Patient advocate
- Delegator
- Supervisor
- Conducting Individual Development and Performance Review (IDPR)

These activities can be categorised under five key components identified at the beginning of the chapter, or under the six core dimensions of healthcare posts detailed in the *NHS KSF* (DH, 2004a), namely communication; personal and people development; health, safety and security; service improvement; quality; and equality and diversity. Examples of day-to-day activities in relation to these headings are presented in Table 1.1.

Furthermore, the DCM has to undertake these activities with full awareness of contemporary and evidence-based modes of clinical practice.

Standards of proficiency and key roles

Preparation for management roles are addressed in pre-registration nursing programmes as identified by the Nursing and Midwifery Council's (NMC) (2004a) *Standards of Proficiency* under the 'care management' domain. This comprises five outcomes for the common foundation programme (usually the first year of the course), and fifteen 'standards of proficiency' for 'entry to the register'. These are reproduced in Box 1.1.

Comparable standards have also been published by the Health Professions Council for allied health professionals such as physiotherapists and dieticians. These standards

Table 1.1 *Components of the healthcare practitioner's roles in the practice setting and how they correspond with NHS KSF 'dimensions'*

Components of nursing	The six core dimensions of the *NHS KSF*	Examples of day-to-day activities of the RN
Clinical practice	• Service improvement • Health, safety and security • Quality	• Quality of care • Skill mix; individual competencies • Recording care • Health education function
Management of care	• Health, safety and security • Equality and diversity • Communication	• Allocating patients according to the practitioner's clinical competence
Education	• Personal and people development	• Teaching students at different levels of learning; and preparing for those about to start placement in your practice setting • Health promotion or patient/relative education as required
Research	• Service improvement • Quality	• Awareness of research findings and current studies related to own practice setting and specialism – nursing and medical • Evidence-based practice
Leadership	• Service improvement • Personal and people development	• Being a role model for all aspects of care • Monitoring standards and managing changes

---

Box 1.1: Standards of proficiency for entry to the register – 'Care management' domain (for pre-registration nursing programmes)

Contribute to the identification of actual and potential risks to patients, clients and their carers, to oneself and to others, and participate in measures to promote and ensure health and safety

- Apply relevant principles to ensure the safe administration of therapeutic substances.
- Use appropriate risk assessment tools to identify actual and potential risks.
- Identify environmental hazards and eliminate and/or prevent where possible.
- Communicate safety concerns to a relevant authority.
- Manage risk to provide care which best meets the needs and interests of patients, clients and the public.

Demonstrate an understanding of the role of others by participating in inter-professional working practice

---

> **Box 1.1: Continued**
>
> - Establish and maintain collaborative working relationships with members of the health and social care team and others.
> - Participate with members of the health and social care team in decision-making concerning patients and clients.
> - Review and evaluate care with members of the health and social care team and others.
> - Take into account the role and competence of staff when delegating work.
> - Maintain one's own accountability and responsibility when delegating aspects of care to others.
> - Demonstrate the ability to co-ordinate the delivery of nursing and healthcare.
>
> *Demonstrate literacy, numeracy and computer skills needed to record, enter, store, retrieve and organise data essential for care delivery*
>
> - Literacy – interpret and present information in a comprehensible manner.
> - Numeracy – accurately interpret numerical data and their significance for the safe delivery of care.
> - Information technology and management – interpret and utilise data and technology, taking account of legal, ethical and safety considerations, in the delivery and enhancement of care.
> - Problem-solving – demonstrate sound clinical decision-making which can be justified even when made on the basis of limited information.
>
> *Source*: Nursing and Midwifery Council (NMC) (2004a)

aim to ensure fitness to practice at the point of registration through the development of knowledge and competence. Furthermore, as part of *The NHS Plan*, the Chief Nursing Officer (CNO) (2002) identified ten key roles for nurses and midwives to improve care delivery, which are as follows:

- Order diagnostic investigations such as pathology tests and X-rays
- Make and receive referrals direct, say, to a therapist or pain consultant
- Admit and discharge patients for specified conditions and within agreed protocols
- Manage patient caseloads, say for diabetes or rheumatology
- Run clinics, say, for ophthalmology or dermatology
- Prescribe medicines and treatments
- Carry out a wide range of resuscitation procedures including defibrillation
- Perform minor surgery and outpatient procedures
- Triage patients using the latest IT to the most appropriate health professional
- Take a lead in the way local health services are organised and run.

These are expanded roles that require further educational preparation beyond the point of registration, and are developed over time in line with service requirements. Key roles have similarly been identified for allied health professionals.

Approaches to organising daily care

In the context of the activities identified in Action point 1.1, as the DCM begins a span of duty, they have to organise the care that their patients will receive. There are a number of ways of organising and delivering care, and within healthcare there is a need to achieve the highest quality care and outcomes taking into account the available resources.

A number of factors shape the adoption of the preferred care delivery methods that individual teams or organisations employ. They include the available skill mix (qualified-unqualified staff ratio – discussed in Chapter 7); the level of supervision and the developmental needs of junior staff and learners. The care delivery method can be eclectic rather than singular, and therefore combined in response to the prevailing circumstances within the span of duty.

Choosing how to organise care

A number of models of care delivery are in existence for the organisation and delivery of patient care. The models address principles such as which member of staff provides care for which patient, and who has responsibility for decision-making and managing the care delivery process. The various models reflect issues such as staffing skill mix, clinical specialty and patient group. Some care delivery models are specific to nursing, and the scope of their application is limited to the institutional setting; while others have relevance for other healthcare practitioners and can be applied within community settings.

Team leader

Within the team approach, there is a skill mix of team members such as a Band 6 registered practitioner, a Band 5 registered practitioner and CSWs. The team is led by a registered practitioner referred to as the team leader; the team collectively provide care for a group of patients during the span of duty. The team leader plans, co-ordinates, monitors, supervises and evaluates the care that is delivered and is responsible for assigning patients based on the competencies of the members within the team. The underlying philosophy of this approach is the achievement of goals and outcomes through collaborative teamwork.

The team approach facilitates the supervision of more junior team members while capitalising on individual expertise and competencies. This approach can also foster staff and patient satisfaction as it supports the delivery of holistic care. The team leader has a fundamental role within this approach and needs to be familiar with the care needs of all of the patients being cared for by their team.

Named nurse

A named, qualified nurse who is responsible for a particular patient's nursing care is known as the named nurse. This method gives the nurse responsibility for, and ensures continuity of care for designated patients. They are responsible for the planning and co-ordination of the patient's nursing care from admission (or before) through to discharge and follow-up, and are actively involved in the delivery of some of that care. Shift patterns such as 12-hour shifts and part-time working can prove challenging to this approach, as continuity of care can be affected for patients. This approach has relevance for short episodes of care within the patient journey, such as that delivered within outpatient departments and day surgery units.

Task allocation

Task allocation, also known as the functional method, is where the organisation of care is based on the division of labour. Tasks are allocated according to the qualification, educational preparation and competence of the healthcare practitioner. The assignment of tasks is predominantly hierarchical in nature, in that a senior practitioner, for example, may manage the unit, while CSWs may be allocated to the less complex skills such as making beds and feeding patients. This approach can be compared to that of an assembly line with the combined interventions of a number of individuals, each of whom has a component part. Within this approach, the DCM can allocate tasks and can easily check if they have been completed as there is a limited margin for overlap.

This approach was prevalent in the mid-twentieth century, although it continues to hold some value for contemporary practice in relation to efficiency, particularly where shortages of staff are experienced. Some specialist areas, such as renal dialysis units and aspects of theatre nursing might utilise this approach, as it lends itself to the technical nature of care delivery and the high patient turnover.

Total care

Total care is also referred to as the case method; within this method, a practitioner is responsible for all aspects of the care for one or more patients, for the duration of the shift. This method is typically used in areas requiring a high level of expertise and intervention such as in ICUs and the community. This approach is patient-focused and encompasses clear lines of accountability. Total care fosters a holistic approach to care delivery; however, it is not considered to be cost-effective with registered practitioners engaging in all aspects of patient care when some of the essential care needs could be met through delegation to CSWs.

Case management

Case management is also known as the care organisation method, in which a named healthcare practitioner assesses a particular patient on first referral or visit, and takes on responsibility for their ongoing care. This method is used in the care of patients with ongoing mental health problems, and those with learning disabilities, in which the practitioner maintains contact with the patient until intervention is no longer required. As the prime manager of the patient's care needs, the DCM arranges and ensures all required care is delivered along the planned pathway.

Primary nursing

Primary nursing encompasses accountability for 24-hour care by one qualified nurse for a group of patients throughout the duration of their hospital stay. Primary nursing is both a philosophy and a system, and is associated with high levels of patient satisfaction. The achievement of primary nursing, however, can be challenging when the primary nurse is away from the practice setting. This method is also resource intensive and its popularity in acute care settings is limited.

Managed care

The managed care method is a multi-disciplinary path of care determined for each patient specific to their medical diagnosis. The path is the critical pattern of events and progress that should be achieved for that patient, from the point of diagnosis to the expected date of discharge. The coordination of the path to ensure that all the actions are carried out by the relevant healthcare practitioners is often completed by an RN.

Key working

There are several interpretations of the term key working, but in the context of the organisation of care, the key working method entails an identified person being charged with defined responsibility towards a specific group of patients. This method has application for use with clients who have learning disabilities and is also utilised within mental health. It has relevance to the community setting, and the scope of the model extends from meeting health care needs to addressing social needs.

Triage

Triage is a process by which a patient is assessed at the point of contact with the healthcare team, to determine the urgency of the health problem and to designate appropriate healthcare resources to attend to the identified problem. Patients are therefore not seen on a 'first come first served' basis, but on the basis of the identified urgency of their health problem. This approach tends to be used in emergency care settings.

Strengths and weaknesses of different ways of organising care

Particular ways of organising care have their advantages, but can also be problematic. A study by Gullick et al. (2004) for instance compared four models of organisation or care, namely patient allocation, team nursing, primary nursing and task allocation. Seventy-eight per cent of respondents taking part in this study expressed a preference for patient allocation with 47 per cent characterising 'responsibility' and 'control' as positive features for this approach.

Action point 1.2 – Advantages and disadvantages of different approaches to organising care

With regard to organisation of care in the practice setting, for each of the following approaches, identify and record two advantages and two likely disadvantages.

Approach	Advantages	Disadvantages
Team leader		
Named nurse		
Task allocation		
Total patient care		
Case management		
Primary nursing		
Managed care		
Key working		
Triage		

For task allocation for instance, Menzies (1960) identified problems with this method of care organisation, describing how it alienates patients from staff, demotivates staff and is counter to the philosophy of holistic care.

The nature of healthcare for many service providers is that it is provided 24 hours per day, 7 days a week, 52 weeks of the year. It is important that the approach adopted is evaluated in relation to a number of key indicators, such as:

- Patient satisfaction (complaints, commendations, patient surveys)
- Family/carer satisfaction (complaints, commendations)

- The achievement of outcomes (clinical audit, quality metrics)
- Cost effectiveness (budget)
- Multi-disciplinary team satisfaction (sickness statistics, morale, staff surveys).

Integrated care pathways

Integrated Care Pathways (ICP) are evidence-based, multi-professional plans of care, treatment and therapy, that provide a structured plan of care and offer a more integrated approach to patient management and the achievement of outcomes. The success of ICPs is dependent upon collaborative teamwork in the development, implementation, monitoring and evaluation of this approach. Healthcare practitioners need to identify evidence-based practice and reach consensus in relation to the patient management requirements for a particular condition, need or speciality. ICPs provide patients with greater opportunities for involvement in their care, as the care they should receive is clearly identified within timelines set out in the ICP.

Integrated record keeping is an integral element of ICPs with all members of the team sharing and documenting within the same record system. ICPs can also feature in-built strategies to monitor patient outcomes in the form of provision for the analysis of variances and clinical audit. They promote a more standardised approach to care delivery that it is advocated, will lead to a reduction in inconsistencies and inequalities in care delivery. Wales (2003) distinguishes ICPs from other approaches to care delivery in that they encompass integral features that record, track and utilise variances to enhance care delivery. ICPs, therefore, are also supportive of the clinical governance agenda.

ICPs, however, can initially be resource intensive to develop in relation to staff time, although long-term benefits include a reduction in time spent on documentation. Some critics of this approach argue that ICPs promote 'cook-book' medicine, reducing professional autonomy and are therefore not conducive to the delivery of individualised care. Conversely, Middleton and Roberts (2000) assert that members of the multi-professional team can opt not to follow the pathway in individual instances where reasonable justification for this deviation can be provided.

ICPs are developed around an agreed time frame that can be expressed in minutes, hours, days or even weeks, depending upon the focus of the pathway. A stroke pathway, for example, may contain distinct phases such as acute care and rehabilitation, with the duration of the pathway expressed in terms of weeks. Interventions can be mapped out in terms of when they should be performed, together with the anticipated outcomes. Table 1.2 provides a simplistic representation of an ICP, key areas of intervention are highlighted in the first column with a time frame included in this instance from pre-operative assessment, through to post-discharge and outpatient follow up. The blank boxes will detail an agreed plan of intervention mapped out against the time frame for the duration of the pathway. Box 1.2 lists key steps that are identified from the literature as being integral to the successful development of an ICP.

Table 1.2 *Exemplar format of an ICP for 'Day Surgery'*

Intervention	Pre-operative Assessment	Day of surgery	Out-Patient Department
Assessments			
Consultations			
Investigations			
Observations			
Medication			
Pain			
Nutrition			
Health education			
Therapy			
Psychosocial			
Discharge planning			

Box 1.2: Key steps in the development of an integrated care pathway

1 Identify a chosen pathway for a medical condition/need/speciality.
2 Configure a multi-professional working group to develop the ICP; this may include representation from other departments, services, sectors, agencies, etc. dependant upon the time frame for the pathway.
3 Obtain examples of ICPs from other organisations.
4 Consider and action the most appropriate strategy in involving patients in the development of the ICP.
5 Select a time-frame for the pathway i.e. pre-operative, rehabilitation etc.
6 Audit current practice to identify both the optimum time frame and interventions for the ICP.
7 Utilise sources of evidence to reach consensus on evidence-based interventions (National Guidelines, National Standards, National Service Frameworks etc.)
8 Agree a time-frame for the ICP and identify outcomes.
9 Develop inclusion/exclusion criteria for the ICP.
10 Identify variances and how they will be monitored.
11 Agree who will co-ordinate the ICP.
12 Provide staff training and pilot the ICP.
13 Undertake audit.
14 Amend the ICP according to the outcomes of the pilot and the audit results.

This section of the chapter has defined what an ICP is and explored the essential features of this approach for care delivery. To apply some of the processes involved in developing an ICP complete Action point 1.3.

 Action point 1.3 – Developing an integrated care pathway

Firstly, identify a patient condition to form the basis for your pathway.

- Select a time frame for your pathway.
- Develop a format for your pathway using the exemplar outlined in Table 1.2.
- Consider the interventions provided by your own discipline and record these at appropriate points within the pathway.
- Consider the interventions provided by members of the multi-professional team and record these at appropriate points within the pathway.
- Identify and record anticipated outcomes for the interventions included within your pathway.

Following completion of Action point 1.3 reflect upon the steps that you have engaged in.

- If you were to develop an ICP, list six challenges that may present themselves in terms of its development.
- For each challenge identify strategies for how you could both prevent this from becoming a problem and also, should it occur, how you can overcome it.

When an ICP has been formulated and documented, it needs to be communicated to all healthcare practitioners who will be involved in the delivery of the identified clinical interventions. Effective communication is essential to the successful achievement of a number of models for the organisation of patient care and will now be explored.

How the DCM communicates day-to-day care

Communication is inevitably the most significant vehicle for exchanging information related to care and treatment. All clinical interventions that healthcare practitioners undertake require effective communication. Care, treatment and illness prevention would be impossible without the DCM and colleagues communicating patient information with each other. The information includes continuous information gathering, deciding on actions and communicating them to healthcare colleagues. Communication is also a crucial element of teamworking, which is examined in Chapter 10.

On a broader level, communication between human beings is essential for both the survival and the development of society. Humans have an instinctive penchant towards gregarity, and Ellis et al. (2003) for instance suggest that the effectiveness and happiness of adults is directly linked to this. In the context of healthcare delivery, effective communication is both a requirement and a necessity.

How communication occurs

Communication can be defined as an interchange between individual and groups to impart and receive information. It is a process in which two or more parties endeavour to make their intentions known and adjust their messages at each step of the interaction, and in effective communication, a common understanding of the messages is shared throughout. Three sets of modes of communication can be identified, namely:

> **a) Written:**   Typed / word-processed, handwritten, emailed, faxed, texted on mobile phone etc
>
> **b) Oral:**   Speaking with an individual or small group face-to-face, speaking by telephone, shouting, video conferencing, lecturing etc
>
> **c) Non-verbal:**   Listening, gestures, posture, tone of voice etc

Oral or spoken communication is generally accompanied by non-verbal messages, which is often a more accurate reflection of the sender's feelings, and is usually easily detected by the receiver.

Thus, the sender of the message, the message itself and the receiver of the message are essential components of communication. In reality, effective communication between two parties entails a number of necessary events, or steps, as illustrated in Figure 1.1. It starts with the thoughts and ideas that one person wishes to impart to another that he formulates and sends. The listener or receiver receives the message, and might decide to respond, whereupon they formulate and send their own message. However, communication can be influenced by various predisposing factors, such as previous experience in similar situations and each person's aims of the communication (see Figure 1.1):

Figure 1.1 indicates that communication comprises several micro steps each of which is a significant component of effective communication.

Figure 1.1   *Events in an effective communication*

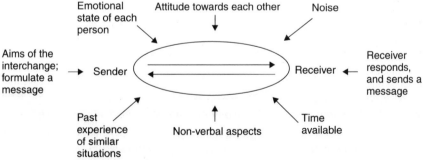

Research on communication in healthcare and healthcare management

Communication in practice settings has been researched for some time. Several studies sponsored by Royal College of Nursing (RCN) were conducted in the 1970s, such as one conducted by Hayward (1975) in relation to the experiences of patients undergoing surgery. Hayward's (1975) study entitled *Information: A Prescription against Pain,* revealed that pre-operative information given to patients led them to require less analgesia post-operatively, become more contented and get discharged from hospital earlier.

Many such studies were conducted in the 1970s and 1980s at a time of raised awareness of the need to base nursing interventions on research. Funds were therefore specifically allocated for these empirical studies. More recent research on communication includes focused areas such as managers' personal skills (e.g. Calpin-Davies, 2000 – detailed in Chapter 2; and Burnard and Morrison, 2005 – related to helping skills).

The DCM's role as communicator

DCMs communicate with several individuals including their subordinates, superiors, peers, medical staff, other healthcare professionals, patients and their families/carers, and social care staff.

Moreover, the directions of communication constitute formal and informal communication. Examples include (see also Figure 1.2):

- **Downward:** Manager discussing with, or instructing a subordinate about what needs to be done, and how
- **Upward:** To provide management with information for decision making
- **Lateral:** Between peers of the same hierarchical level – for information sharing/negotiation
- **Diagonal:** Between individuals or departments at different hierarchical levels – for requesting and giving information, for instance

Scammell (1990) suggests that the specific reasons for effective and efficient communications by managers are to:

- establish and disseminate goals of the enterprise;
- develop plans for their achievement;
- organise human and other resources in the most effective and efficient way;
- select, develop and appraise members of the organisation;
- lead, direct and motivate members of the organisation; and
- control performance.

Figure 1.2 *Directions of communication between staff nurses and ward sisters*

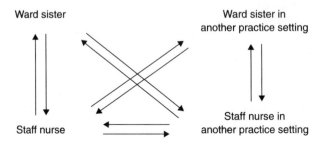

Some communication can take place in challenging circumstances such as when a complaint has been received, or when breaking bad news. However, instances of communication that are specifically management communication include:

a) Delegation of duties
b) Arranging and conducting meetings
c) Conducting IDPR
d) Team-building exercises
e) Report writing
f) Negotiation
g) Making presentations
h) Staff interviews, for example, for recruitment and problem-solving
i) Motivational activities
j) Counselling.

Going by the above list, and the various managerial roles of the DCM discussed in the next chapter, it is obvious that all management functions include communication. The mechanics of the first item in the above list, that is, delegation of duties is now explored as an example of how each of these avenues or functions comprises several facets.

Delegation

An essential responsibility and function of the DCM is to delegate the work that needs to be carried out to appropriate members of the healthcare team. Curtis and Nicholl (2004:26) suggest that delegation is becoming increasingly important because of changes, such as:

- The falling number of nurses
- Issues around skill mix
- Restructuring how care is delivered
- The expanding role of nurses.

The American Nurses Association and National Council of State Boards of Nursing (2005) jointly define delegation as a process to direct another person to perform tasks and activities. They highlight, however, that authority and responsibility for the performance of an activity can be transferred, but accountability for the outcome is retained. The following points should be considered by the DCM to ensure effective delegation:

- Ultimate accountability for all work rests with the registered healthcare practitioner, and therefore what to delegate to non-registered staff needs careful consideration.
- Delegation can provide subordinates with opportunities to learn, and can support their career development.
- Staff morale can improve through the responsibility that goes with delegation.
- All delegation involves some risk, but can be minimised by measured coaching and effective supervision.
- Despite careful preparation, mistakes can occur, and the DCM should be able to learn from them, rather than stop delegating.

The various stages for effective delegation are as follows:

1. Assessment of tasks that need to be completed	2. Matching tasks to compe- tencies of delegates	3. Assign- ing tasks	4. Tasks are completed by delegates	5. Supervising and monitoring task completion	6. Evalua- tion and feedback as appropriate

It should be noted that steps 4 and 5 are usually undertaken simultaneously rather than as separate entities. Some managers believe: 'If you want a job done properly, do it yourself', which equates to a 'reluctance to let go' (Scammell, 1990:42). As part of the delegation process the manager needs to consider the importance of the task and the implications if it is not completed properly or on time. The manager can utilise a number of strategies to support the delegation process such as coaching and a contingency plan should any problems be experienced.

Communication is fundamental to all aspects of the role of the DCM. Each management function can be unpacked to ascertain the various component parts. These can be defined, the reasons for the communication examined, the issues surrounding each explored, and how they can be operationalised ascertained. For instance, arranging and conducting meetings can include:

- Types of meetings
- Membership and terms of reference
- Functions of meetings
- Mechanics of meetings
- Seating positions and impact on the meeting's outcomes
- Reasons for attending meetings
- Chairing a meeting – managing time, the process, the people
- Involving group members in the meeting
- Constructing task subgroups
- Communicating outcomes.

Communication problems

A further important perspective to consider in relation to communication is how it can be improved. There are a number of 'barriers' to communication and the various reasons for communication breakdown need to be considered to enable the DCM to be an effective communicator.

 Action point 1.4 – Communication breakdown

Think of a situation where a communication breakdown has occurred within your practice setting. This could be communication between colleagues, or between a healthcare practitioner and a patient. Consider the reason/s for this breakdown of communication and identify ways in which this could have been avoided.

Communication breakdown could mean that the individual feels that necessary information (the message) being imparted was markedly misunderstood or misinterpreted. Communication can be classified as effective, ineffective and persuasive. Furthermore, as Yoder-Wise (2003) suggests, poor communication can lead to conflict, which is a reality in organisations, but which presents opportunities for change and progress, as discussed in Chapter 4.

Different forms of communication have application in different situations ranging from basic to more specialist communication skills. Scammell (1990:14) identifies a useful range of communication skills that are illustrated by a communication continuum, starting with primary communications such as in initial contacts with others, to specialist communication such as secondary counselling. Secondary counselling constitutes specialised communication skills that are developed over several years of training and experience. It includes utilisation of particular communication frameworks such as Heron's (1989) 'Six-category intervention analysis', which constitutes a model of counselling with six possible interactions that are started by the initiator of the communication. These are:

Authoritative interventions:

- **Prescriptive:**   Give advice on correct action to take
- **Informative:**   Give concrete factual information
- **Confrontational:** Challenging perceptions expressed

Facilitative interventions:

- **Supportive:**   Accepting the person, giving time and reflective learning
- **Cathartic:**   Enabling to express emotions
- **Catalytic:**   Being as neutral and as unbiased as possible

Effective communication underpins all aspects of management and leadership and is an essential skill for the DCM. Communication in the context of teamwork is further discussed in Chapter 10.

Guidelines for the effective organisation of care

- Organise daily care delivery based on the patient's healthcare needs
- Allocate patients to staff with the appropriate clinical skills to ensure the best use of skill mix
- Ensure all plans and actions are communicated fully, appropriately and effectively to all concerned
- As the DCM, delegate duties responsibly and in line with professional accountability
- Monitor and supervise duties that you delegate to ensure that they are completed to the required standard.

Chapter summary

This chapter started by examining the broader context of care management, which includes a range of factors related to the prevailing social context in which care and treatment are delivered. This included exploration of:

- the prevailing social context of healthcare provision such as working as a DCM in contemporary healthcare, with current government policies guiding how healthcare organisations are to respond to the healthcare needs of society;
- the roles and functions of the qualified healthcare practitioner as a DCM, including micro level exploration of the roles and specific activities that are undertaken in the course of daily duties.
- approaches to organising care delivery, including integrated care pathways, together with an assessment of the strengths and weaknesses of each method discussed; and
- the reasons, nature and modes of communication utilised by DCMs, which included the role of communication in management and leadership, effective communication, types of management communication, followed by problems of communication.

Strong and effective management and leadership are required at all levels within health and social care. The DCM needs to have an understanding of the context within which contemporary healthcare is delivered and to be able to translate this to their role within their individual practice setting. The various aspects of management and leadership will now be explored in Chapters 2 and 3 respectively.

TWO Managing effectively – theories, roles and styles

Introduction

The DCM has a pivotal role in ensuring delivery of the highest standards of care and treatment whilst also ensuring optimal use of available resources. Having ascertained in Chapter 1 the various options available to the DCM for organising the care of patients and communicating effectively, this chapter now examines the theories, roles and styles that underpin effective management in the practice setting.

Chapter objectives

On completion of this chapter you will be able to:

- ascertain the specific day-to-day managerial activities that the DCM engages in;
- recognise the importance of organisational structure, differentiate between types of structure and identify how they influence organisational performance;
- distinguish between the key terms manager and management, and comprehend the various theories and styles of management that the DCM can draw on;
- identify specific management roles that the manager fulfils, and explore the personal qualities required to be a successful clinical manager;
- identify where management of care fits in within the larger organisational and management structures of healthcare organisations; and
- demonstrate knowledge and understanding of how to apply significant theories of management to practice settings, and thereby develop your personal managerial skills.

The day-to-day activities of the duty clinical manager

The end of the twentieth century saw varied questions and concerns raised about healthcare management. In particular, these were related to the amount of money being spent on health services. Yet scientific advances will always uncover new and more effective ways of treating illnesses, which in turn tends to cumulatively increase the expenses of healthcare organisations. The quality of care provision has also latterly been under the spotlight. Effective management is therefore an imperative to ensure these concerns are addressed.

At times managers might appear to be engrossed primarily in administrative duties such as 'doing the paperwork', or they might seem to be engaged in meetings within or outside the department. At other times, they might appear to do no more than ensure that their employees are conducting their key roles correctly, and intervene only when problems are anticipated or arise. Nevertheless, as the DCM may be the healthcare practitioner or the ward manager/team leader in charge of a span of duty, they have to balance their care delivery duties, with those of care management.

 Action point 2.1 – Clinical management activities

This action point can be undertaken in small groups, in pairs or individually.

i   Identify and write down *all* 'real life' day-to-day management or managerial activities undertaken by the DCM in your workplace, and issues dealt with, over:

- a particular span of duty
- a 24-hour period
- a one week period
- a period of one month.

This includes dealing with routine as well as with unexpected events during different spans of duty.

ii Now list the reasons why you think managers engage in each of these activities.

In addition to the list of managerial activities that you have compiled, there are likely to be other activities undertaken when considered over longer periods of time. Your list of managerial duties might include many of those listed in the left hand column of Table 2.1. This table combines a range of management activities identified by RNs on management courses, and by finalist pre-registration student nurses separately, and extracts key components of day-to-day management of care and treatment, and management roles.

The day-to-day managerial activities of the DCM identified in Table 2.1 are key management components that are extrapolated and identified as managerial roles in the right hand column of Table 2.1. These managerial components form the basis of effective management in the practice setting. Back in the earlier part of the twentieth century, Fayol (1949) conducted a much-quoted study that identified management activities (or functions) as planning, organising, commanding, co-ordinating and controlling (feedback), which was claimed to have universal relevance.

Although the 12 managerial roles in Table 2.1 are identified as discrete activities, in reality they are all interlinked to form the overall picture of the DCM's management activities in today's practice settings. They represent quite an accurate reflection of contemporary roles of DCMs. Further details of components that each role represents are presented in Table 2.2.

This discussion on the activities of DCMs focuses attention on the practical aspects of their role during a typical span of duty, but their line manager would have ongoing responsibility and accountability for the practice setting. There are of course various other ways of categorising management activities. Drucker (1979), for instance,

Table 2.1 *The day-to-day managerial activities of the DCM, as identified by RNs and finalist pre-registration student nurses*

Managerial activities identified by RNs and finalist pre-registration student nurses	Managerial components or roles
Workload management Doing the off-duty/Self-rostering Staffing levels and skill-mix Dealing with staff shortages/crises Staff interviews and recruitment Identifying annual leave	*Human resource manager*
Sickness management Staff morale issues Acting as staff advocate	*Promoter of staff welfare*
Bed management Managing space i.e. extra beds/patients on trolleys	*Capacity manager*
Budgeting Ensuring resources are available e.g. equipment Collecting statistics	*Effectiveness and efficiency monitor*
Delegation (of duties) Arranging and attending meetings	*Planner and communicator*
Dealing with personality clashes, conflict between staff Bleep holder, deal with crisis Liaising with other agencies e.g. education	*Decision-maker and problem-solver*
Dealing with/preventing complaints from staff/patients /their relatives Involved in audits Other clinical governance activities	*Quality assuror*
Dealing with child protection issues Risk management Ensuring safety of patients, staff, etc., deal with accidents	*Guardian of health and safety*
Disciplining and grievance	*Policy enforcer*
Allocating study time/training Staff training needs and statutory training; education programme Monitoring mandatory training Handling and moving; CPD, Fire – regular updates Appraisals (IDPR)	*Staff trainer and educator*
Hands-on clinical care	*Clinician and practice developer*
Giving information Mentor/supervise junior RNs	*Leader and team worker*

identifies five 'basic operations' in the work of the manager as setting objectives, organising, motivating and communicating, measuring and developing people. Alternatively, Reynolds (2003) maintains that managers manage people and their activities, resources, information and themselves. Both examples illustrate how

Table 2.2 *Brief details of each managerial role*

Managerial role	Further details or components
Human resource manager	Recruitment, staff retention, motivating the team, dealing with performance issues
Promoter of staff welfare	Knowledge of facilities and support that staff can draw on
Capacity manager	Ensures adequately skilled staff provide and perform clinical interventions effectively
Effectiveness and efficiency monitor	Monitors use of resources, both human and non-human resources
Planner and communicator	Communicates, delegates and negotiates plans and changes
Decision-maker and problem-solver	Makes decisions at operational level; pre-empt/solve problems; conflict manager
Quality assuror	Monitors informally and formally the quality of care provided to patients; ensures equality and supports diversity
Guardian of health and safety	Ensures health and safety regulations, ethical guidelines and professional codes are adhered to
Policy enforcer	Ensures clinical policies and guidelines are adhered to; devises/ adapts guidelines as necessary
Staff trainer/educator	Identifies, contributes to and monitors team members' professional development and learning
Clinician and practice developer	Manages change and innovations
Leader and team worker	Leader of the team; maintains team cohesiveness, which can be multi-professional

grouping information into fewer categories of more generalised terms causes loss of detail of the multiple and complex activities that the DCM engages in during a span of duty, which then need to be interpreted and applied.

It is essential to appreciate that when engaged in the management activities (or managerial roles) that emerged from Action point 2.1, these are undertaken in the context of the overall healthcare organisation where the healthcare practitioner works.

Management and organisations

Table 2.1 identified the activities of the DCM as many and varied. So how are the terms manager and management defined?

Managers and management

Most definitions of the terms manager and management refer to the activities and competencies of managers. For instance, Stewart (1997:3) defines a manager as 'someone who gets things done through other people'. Armstrong (2006) suggests that a manager is someone whose main job is to organise their junior colleagues' time within an organisation in order to pursue the objectives of the organisation. In today's healthcare organisations, a manager is an employee who has been appointed specifically to ensure that the objectives of their span of remit are achieved effectively and efficiently. The DCM is a registered healthcare practitioner with appropriate knowledge and skills, who therefore decides and prioritises the specific tasks or activities that need to be performed within a span of duty, and then ensures that they have been performed competently by appropriately skilled personnel.

Managers often work in collaboration with other managers, who are either of similar status, more senior or more junior than them. A group of managers could comprise a management team, which might include clinical directors, a general manager, modern matrons and consultant nurses.

According to Drucker (1979), management, in the context of a management team, is 'a multi-purpose organ' that manages a business and its employees as individuals and teams, with the aim of accomplishing the goals of the organisation. The analogy of an 'organ' in Drucker's definition could be seen to imply that management is a live and dynamic entity that can grow and enable others to grow, or could be affected by problematic issues that need resolving. Clinical management comprises a team of qualified healthcare practitioners, who fulfil the functions identified in Table 2.1, which includes being a clinician. Therefore, the term management can be defined as a team of appropriately qualified individuals who engage in multiple activities aimed at achieving the goals of the organisation effectively and efficiently.

Each healthcare trust is an organisation in its own right, and healthcare interventions are carried out in the context of the particular organisation's specific function, which is to support the local population's healthcare needs. Organisations can span generations, and an individual employee may opt to leave at some point, but the organisation itself is likely to endure and outlive all individual employees by many years. Therefore most organisations are very likely to continue existing long after current and subsequent managers have served their term and left for other posts or even retired.

The healthcare trust as an organisation

The aims and objectives of the healthcare organisation would normally be specified in the Business Plan, along with its Mission Statement. A healthcare organisation is a service organisation, and organisations can therefore be distinguished in terms of two generic groups: public sector organisations and private enterprise organisations. The distinction between the two is that public sector organisations do not have profit as their goal, they are 'owned' by taxpayers and ratepayers, and their main aim is to provide a service that is concerned with the well-being of individuals in the community in the particular catchment area. Private organisations tend to be owned and financed by individuals, partners, shareholders, and the main aim is of a commercial nature, that is, financial profit. However, the boundary between public and private sector is blurred to some extent with the prevalence of internal markets within healthcare and the advent of Foundation Trusts.

Thus, organisations vary according to the nature of the work they undertake. For example, contrasting a school with a car manufacturer, or a hospital with a public library, shows that each has distinct functions. These functions determine the people skills they require, how simple or complex they are, their size in the context of their output, the number of people they employ, and also the extent to which they utilise technology.

To achieve the aims of the organisation, a managing director, or in an NHS trust, a chief executive is appointed. The chief executive, in turn, is accountable to the chairperson of the appropriate trust Board, and in healthcare, to the Strategic Health Authority and then ultimately to the Secretary of State for Health. This is likely to change as NHS trusts move rapidly towards achieving 'NHS Foundation Trust' status that entails decentralisation of public services and devolution of decision-making from central government control to local organisations and communities so that they are more responsive to the needs and wishes of the local population (DH, 2007c).

The activities and performance of NHS Foundation Trusts are however regularly checked by 'Monitor' which is the independent regulator of Foundation Trusts. Monitor is responsible for authorising, monitoring and regulating Foundation Trusts to ensure that they are well-managed and financially strong so that they can deliver 'excellent' healthcare for patients. Monitor has the powers to intervene in the running of NHS Foundation Trusts in the event of failings in their healthcare standards or other aspects of their activities, which amount to a significant breach of their terms of authorisation.

The structure of organisations

In addition to the building, or the complex of buildings that house a healthcare organisation, its staffing structure constitutes all individuals employed in it, and the precise division of work, that is the allocation of individual tasks and responsibilities to each employee. This entails establishing a structure of senior and junior staff with clearly demarcated duties, responsibilities and span of control, and may be hierarchical in nature. It also incorporates reporting relationships within the organisation, and the pattern of relationships between different posts and different employees, as well as the co-ordination of their activities that are directed towards achieving the organisation's goals and objectives. The hierarchical structure of employees is the mechanism through which the activities of the organisation are allocated and monitored.

Within the structure of the organisation, various channels of communication are established to ensure they are effective. Team brief, staff meetings, bulletins and email communications are just a few examples of modes of communication.

Organisational structures consist of a number of inherent common dimensions such as grouping of functions into sections and departments, and the objectives of each of these departments need to be consistent with and contribute to those of the organisation as a whole. The work that needs to be done has to be clearly defined, and should be divided up appropriately amongst employees. Consequently, this constitutes the integration of the efforts and full participation of each individual employee. Motivation of staff through systems of appraisal and reward should also be established and implemented.

The allocation of individual tasks and responsibilities also comprises job specialisation and job definition. The degree of specialisation required to achieve the objectives of the organisation has to be delineated, and in nursing as well as in other healthcare professions generally, there is increasing specialisation and demarcation of responsibilities that change and blur roles, and influence the nature of employees' roles within the organisation.

Each employee's function in the organisational structure is important, as this impacts on productivity, morale and job satisfaction. Another crucial factor is the frame of reference that takes account of the 'people factor', such as appropriate leadership and management styles. However, a good structure does not singularly guarantee success, as appropriate systems of work need to be in place, and effectiveness needs to be monitored and evaluated regularly.

Hierarchical levels in the organisation

Varying levels of hierarchy exists within organisations. This could comprise a pyramidal structure, as illustrated in Figure 2.1.

Action point 2.2 – The hierarchy in your practice setting

- Draw a diagram identifying the staffing structure within your team.
- How many levels of command are there, and what are the possible advantages and disadvantages of these particular levels of hierarchy?
- Do you consider the management structure and levels of command within your practice setting to be appropriate?
- What management structure do you consider to be ideal?

The current hierarchy of different levels of employees in any particular practice setting, or organisation could be functioning effectively, but due to ongoing changes influenced by internal and external factors (see Chapter 6 for more detail) flaws could appear, and therefore the existing management structure needs to be regularly reviewed.

Variations in the number of levels of management in the organisation and each manager's span of control can influence the effectiveness with which responsibilities are fulfilled. With pyramidal structures for instance, clinical managers might choose to devolve certain functions to more junior members of staff. For example, rather than personally undertaking IDPR for all staff working within the team, the clinical manager might devolve those for CSWs to other senior healthcare practitioners. However, there could be a danger that steep pyramidal structures could result in ineffective communication and relationships between the next-but-one level of

Figure 2.1 *Pyramidal management structure*

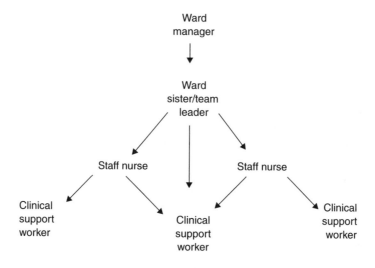

Figure 2.2 *Flatter management structure*

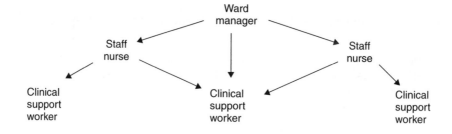

management, which in turn could lead to misrepresentations and misunderstandings, such as when changes to work conditions are proposed.

Flatter structures

Flatter management structures could resolve some of the issues related to pyramidal structures, and enable the organisation to meet the need for individual employees to achieve more autonomy, and to feel 'personal growth' within their posts.

Using management theories

Numerous published theories of management are available to choose from, but before examining specific ones, it is pertinent to establish what a theory is and what the purposes of theories are. All human actions are based on some theory, that is, certain assumptions, hypotheses and generalisations. Theories tend to determine our prediction that if we do *a*, then *b* will occur, that is, it incorporates a 'cause and effect' type of relationship. A theory is a structure of ideas that seeks to explain a phenomenon that may be based around a number of principles.

Consequently, management theories (discussed next) also aim to fulfil such functions as describing, predicting and explaining the wherewithal of management of practice settings. So, on which management theories can DCMs base their management functions? The theories available could be grouped under 'conventional management' theories and 'managerial role' theory. There are four main conventional management theories, namely the classical theory, human relations theory, systems theory and contingency theory. A subsequent theory referred to as post-modern theory has been mooted more recently.

Conventional management theories

The classical approach

The classical approach is one of the earliest management theories, but one that can still be easily observed in bureaucratic organisations today. According to this theory, which was known as 'scientific management' in its early years, managers guide the organisation to improve efficiency. It constitutes the notion that if a formal structure is firmly established with regard to exactly who does specific jobs, the technical skills they need to have to fulfil the job requirements and a set of detailed procedures that they need to follow to do so, then the organisation would function effectively and efficiently. The formal structure is designed accordingly with the aim being the achievement of the organisation's goals. It includes a clear hierarchy of staff, with formal intra-organisational relationships, clear division of work and definition of duties and responsibilities, as well as established rules and procedures for various activities.

The scientific management theory was originally advocated by Taylor (1856–1917). It comprises:

- concern with improvements that are designed to increase productivity;
- one 'best working method' to do a job, and this can be done by breaking jobs into discrete tasks and 'one best way' to perform each task;
- provision of monetary incentives as a motivator for high levels of output;
- making management a science by systematic selection, training and development of employees;
- co-operation with workers to ensure work is carried out in the prescribed way; and
- a clear division of work and responsibility between managers and workers.

This management approach was later referred to as the 'bureaucratic' method wherein employment is also based on technical qualification and skills. Some of the main features of the bureaucratic method are:

- specialisation in specific duties and responsibilities;
- a clear hierarchy of authority and precise stratification (as in the army, or a factory production line); and
- specific relatively stable rules that are designed to provide efficient operation including clearly laid down appeal procedures against management decisions.

Table 2.3 *Strengths and weaknesses of the scientific approach of management*

Strengths of the scientific approach	Weaknesses of the scientific approach
✓ Better quality of management decisions	✗ Bureaucratic i.e. structured rules, regulations, templates
✓ Reduced employee turnover	✗ Managers ensure that rules are adhered to
✓ Less sickness and absenteeism	✗ May lack flexibility
✓ Fewer accidents	✗ Can be impersonal
✓ Better labour relations	

The likely strengths and weaknesses of the scientific approach are highlighted in Table 2.3.

However, as with the scientific approach, there are also weaknesses in bureaucratic methods, including:

- over-emphasis on rules and regulations that can stifle growth and initiative, and lead to failure, frustration and conflict and stereotyped behaviours; and
- neglect of the employee's aspirations.

However, although scientific management methods can be applied to clinical management, the theory tends to overlook the interpersonal needs and interactions between employees, and their individual views on the functioning of the organisation. The method therefore often proves unacceptable to the employee and often to managers. Subsequent theories of management, such as the human relations approach, emerged to overcome this major weakness in the classical approach by incorporating the personal and social experiences of individual workers.

The human relations approach

A landmark in the development of the human relations approach was the findings of the momentous Hawthorne experiments in the Western Electric Company in the United States during the period 1924 to 1932. One of the findings of the experiments was that productivity (or the amount of work done during a particular shift) increased when people worked in groups, especially if these groups were self-selected. This approach consequently takes account of some of the psychological and social needs of the employees of the organisation.

The human relations approach is also referred to as the 'behavioural' or 'informal approach', and later developments of this approach include neo-human relations theories, which includes concepts and theories developed by Maslow (1987), Herzberg (1974), McGregor (1987) and others. The work of these authors has direct impact on staff motivation because of their focus on human needs as discussed in Chapter 10 in relation to teamwork.

The human relations theory is clearly the most appropriate approach for managing healthcare staff, primarily because the whole ethos of health services is founded on caring and promoting the holistic well-being of people. Some of the ways in which the DCM could effectively implement this approach are presented in Box 2.1.

Box 2.1: Ways in which the human relations theory could be effectively applied by the DCM

- Taking into account each individual member of staff's personal prospects in relation to their post e.g. personal and professional development needs, forming new alliances, etc.
- Attending to social factors by encouraging staff to socialise during short beaks, etc.
- Encouraging groups of staff to work as a team, rather than as separate individuals.
- Monitoring how new members of staff are 'fitting in' with the existing team.
- Showing an appropriate level of interest in the employee's family, birthdays, wedding, new baby, etc.
- Maintaining a structure that provides sufficient availability of clinical supervision and peer support for individual members of staff.

 Action point 2.3 – Implementing the human relations approach

Think of various instances when managers who you know demonstrate a human relations approach by adopting features like those identified in Box 2.1.

How feasible it is to implement all these features depends on several other factors. For instance, certain provisions might not be in place due to resource constraints, levels of employees' motivation and their knowledge and competence. It could also be said that it is difficult to please all staff, all of the time. These issues will be explored further under the management of change (in Chapter 6). However, dedicating excessive time using the human relations approach at the expense of scientific methods could also negatively affect productivity.

Additionally, new mechanical equipment and electronic medical devices that facilitate healthcare workers' daily duties have evolved over the years, with new ones emerging all the time requiring regular re-learning by staff. The 'systems approach' to management takes into account the utilisation of these necessary aids.

The systems approach

The systems approach to management recognises organisations as comprising of a number of systems and sub-systems, and subsumes the advantageous aspects of classical and human relations' approaches. This approach sees organisations as (i) open systems, with multiple channels of interaction internally and with the broader external environment; and (ii) socio-technical system, which recognises the relationship between social and technical variables within the organisation. The socio-technical system not only heeds the increasing need to use new technologies to accelerate and improve the quality of organisational outcomes, but also advocates heeding the effect this might have on individual employees.

The systems approach is clearly visible in practice settings where medical technology is required for clinical interventions, diagnostic technologies that enable a wide range of pathology laboratory investigations and those that enable results to be communicated more speedily to clinical staff. In other team structures, non-medical practitioners can be involved in undertaking minor surgical or endoscopic procedures. The recognition of the role that these facilitative devices play to support the delivery of care, treatment and communication by managers form the basis of this approach.

The contingency approach

The three management theories briefly discussed above evolved over several decades in the order presented, but the more recent and widely adopted theory is referred to as the 'contingency approach'. The contingency approach, which is also referred to as situational management, stipulates that there is no one optimum state in an organisation, and therefore the management approach utilised, and its success, is dependent (or 'contingent') upon the nature of the task that needs to be undertaken or situation dealt with, at a particular point in time, and under prevailing environmental circumstances.

The contingency approach therefore comprises the belief that there is no one best and universally applicable management theory as there are a large number of variables and situational factors that have an influence on organisational performance. It is seen as an 'if–then' form of relationship. 'If' a particular situation exists, 'then' the scientific approach might be the most appropriate, such as, if a newly qualified healthcare practitioner is learning new clinical procedures, then he or she must follow the trust's procedure or clinical guidelines. In other situations the human relations approach might be more appropriate, such as when dealing with a patient who has expressed concern regarding the standard of care received. Consequently, over particular periods of time, the DCM might well choose to use an appropriate combination of the three approaches. Box 2.2 presents a summary of conventional theories of management.

Box 2.2: Summary of conventional theories of management

Classical management theory   Involves having:

- clearly defined goals
- formal hierarchical management structures
- common procedures and policies
- minimal or no consideration of employees' views.

Human relations theory   Incorporates consideration of:

- social factors in the work setting
- formal groups and emerging sub-groups
- appropriate leadership
- personal matters.

Box 2.2: Continued

Systems theory	Builds on:

- classical and human relations approaches, and further develops them
- up-to-date technological aids
- the organisation vis-à-vis its external environment.

Contingency theory   Stipulates that:

- there is no one best management theory
- the management approach taken is based on the nature of the situation at that point in time.

The post-modern approach

Beyond conventional management theories, the post-modern approach to management is advocated. This approach is based on post-modern philosophies and beliefs about society in general (e.g. Petersen and Bunton, 1997; Rolfe, 1999), which suggests that every situation requires a rethink of all alternative approaches or avenues available every time as there could well be other unprecedented, or more than one appropriate, acceptable and effective approach to countenance a situation.

For instance in healthcare, the NHS III (2007a) suggests that 'lean' thinking as a management system refers to the least wasteful way to provide healthcare, which also maximises the use of resources, and reduces delays. Castle (2007) suggests that lean methods are implemented by top level managers by devolving quality assurance and various other responsibilities to teams of employees who are skilled in a variety of tasks, and by reduced individual specialisation.

Managerial roles theory

This section focuses on management theories from another angle, which is that of managerial roles theory. Table 2.2 identifies 12 managerial roles of the clinical manager, which are illustrated in Figure 2.3. These roles reflect a comprehensive approach to management in healthcare.

Another managerial roles theory was proposed earlier by Mintzberg (1990) who suggested ten key role areas as follows:

1.	**Figurehead**	Represents the practice setting formally
2.	**Liaison**	Deals with peers and outsiders in order to exchange work-related information
3.	**Leader**	Staffs the practice setting and motivates employees
4.	**Monitor**	Gathers and interprets necessary information
5.	**Disseminator**	Passes on to subordinates information not otherwise available
6.	**Spokesperson**	Passes on information to external agencies

7. **Entrepreneur**   Initiates change and innovations
8. **Disturbance handler**   Intervenes when disruptions occur
9. **Resource allocator**   Decides where and how resources will be deployed
10. **Negotiator**   Deals with outsiders whose consent and co-operation is required by the practice setting

Mintzberg's ten-role theory is therefore an alternative framework that the DCMs can utilise to analyse and fulfil their management functions in practice settings.

Figure 2.3 *The managerial roles of clinical managers*

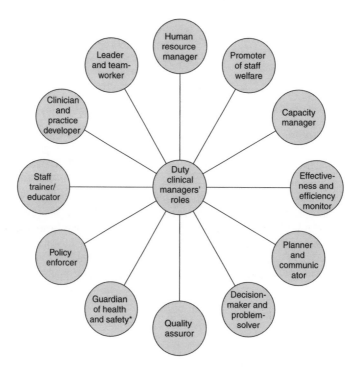

 Action point 2.4 – Your own managerial roles

Recall recent managerial tasks that you have undertaken, and consider how these relate to the managerial roles in clinical management identified in Figure 2.3.

- Using the format below, examine specific ways in which you get directly involved in each of these managerial roles.
- After you have completed the second column, rate the extent of your skill and self-confidence with each role from 1 to 5, where 1 represents low skill and self-confidence and 5 represents high.
- How effective do you feel in each of the roles you undertake?

Action point 2.4 – Continued

- Ask your line manager how effective they believe you to be in each of these roles.
- Consider self-development opportunities to equip you to become more effective in each of these roles.

MANAGEMENT ROLES	My specific involvement in management roles	Skill rating	Self-confidence rating
Human resource manager			
Promoter of staff welfare			
Capacity manager			
Effectiveness and efficiency monitor			
Planner and communicator			
Decision-maker and problem-solver			
Quality assuror			
Guardian of health and safety			
Policy enforcer			
Staff trainer/educator			
Clinician and practice developer			
Leader and team-worker			

The actions suggested above might have overlapped to a fair extent with that of Action point 2.1, but will nonetheless have enabled you to identify your own areas of strength as a manager, as well as those of deficit, and those in which you wish your management role to develop further.

Styles of management

In addition to theories of management, another dimension to managing people is the notion of management styles. The word 'style' refers to the characteristic or manner in which the person expresses himself in social situations, and therefore performs his managerial tasks, and this also applies to the DCM. It incorporates how managers, being in positions of authority, conduct themselves and their tasks towards their juniors, to the general public and to their seniors.

One of the most prominent perspectives on styles of management is advocated by Blake and McCanse (1991) who identified the manager's style as reflecting 'concern for people' that is, their employees, or 'concern for productivity' that is, the amount of work completed. High 'concern for people' is consistent with a democratic style, as opposed to an autocratic style and the human relations approach to management. High concern for productivity indicates that the manager performs his tasks with the principal focus being on how much work gets done, which is largely related to the classical approach.

Another popular style of management was advocated even earlier by Odiorne (1979) as well as Drucker (1979), which is known as 'Management by objectives' (MBO), and directly affects contemporary management in healthcare. In this style of management, the manager endeavours to juxtapose the organisation's objectives to those of the individual employee's, along with the latter's development needs. Odiorne (1979) described MBO as a mechanism whereby a manager and each employee jointly identify goals that are common to the employee and to the organisation, and define the individual's major areas of responsibility in terms of results. MBO is consequently founded on (i) defining specific areas of responsibility, setting objectives and targets, and criteria of performance and the continual review and appraisal of results; and (ii) the professional development needs of the employee.

MBO has been widely used in both private and public sectors and focuses on people's strengths enabling their further development, rather than concentrating on their weaknesses. When reviewing performance, the manager concentrates on the tasks that the employee has completed, but does not treat completion or non-completion as a feature of their character or personality. The focus is on the achievement of objectives.

Consequently, the MBO style of management incorporates the use of IDPR. However, the individual employee's objectives and targets are not imposed but established and agreed through discussion between them and their line manager. Thus, within agreed limits and the policies of the organisation, employees are given some freedom of action to decide how best to achieve their objectives and targets. MBO can be contrasted with the more autocratic management style that is based on direction and control.

One possible drawback of MBO is that it could focus too much on the job and reflect the scientific management approach; another is that it also assumes that there will be complete alignment between individuals and the organisation's goals.

Applied to healthcare organisations, MBO tends to figure in the organisation's Business Plan in the form of strategic and operational objectives. Annual IDPR for healthcare practitioners working in practice settings in the NHS is specified as the skills framework and review in the *NHS KSF* (DH, 2004a). This document provides a structure that directly links the healthcare organisation's skill needs for the achievement of corporate objectives with the individual employee's self-determined responsibilities and professional development needs. Accordingly, employees need to identify their competence and development needs in six core dimensions, namely:

1 Communication
2 Personal and people development
3 Health, safety and security
4 Service improvement
5 Quality
6 Equality and diversity.

There are further 'specific dimensions' identified, along with specified levels for each dimension, that correspond with *Agenda for Change* (DH, 2004c) pay bands. The *NHS KSF* is a fully structured framework for facilitating performance reviews, and includes the requirement to develop personal and professional development plans.

The qualities and personal skills of healthcare managers

On examining theories and styles of management that the DCM could adopt in their practice setting, it becomes obvious that personality and personal qualities are also important ingredients of how they are perceived by those they interact with, and manage.

Calpin-Davies (2000) reports on a study that explored the key characteristics and the necessary personal skills of nurse managers. Her findings are summarised in Box 2.3. Additionally, Calpin-Davies (2000) suggests that the nurse manager should also be able to self-manage, and supports Covey's (1992) suggestion that

---

Box 2.3: Key characteristics and personal skills of nurse managers

Key characteristics of nurse managers

- Being service oriented
- Radiating positive energy
- Believing in other people
- Leading balanced professional lives
- Seeing professional life as an adventure
- Being synergistic
- Exercising professional self-renewal

Personal skills of nurse managers

- Communication skills
- Ability to motivate people
- Ability to influence others
- Adaptability and ability to respond positively to change, both planned and unplanned

managers should also develop the 'seven habits' or characteristics of highly effective people, which are:

1 be proactive – planning ahead as opposed to merely reacting to events;
2 begin with the end in mind – determine the outcomes in full prior to deciding on the strategies to be used for achieving them;
3 put first things first – prioritising what needs doing;
4 think win/win – being aware of situations that warrant mutual benefits;
5 seek first to understand, and then to be understood – use of empathy;
6 synergise with others – developing two-way communication and negotiating; and
7 sharpen the saw – adequate rest and relaxation leading to better functioning.

Box 2.4 summarises, the personal qualities of the successful DCM.

Box 2.4: Qualities of the successful DCM

- Has good social skills
- Shows understanding
- Communicates effectively
- Is creative
- Emotionally resilient
- Self-aware
- Solves problems
- Proactive planner
- Has command of basic facts/knowledgeable

- Forward thinking
- Lifelong learner
- Able to motivate
- Articulate
- Nurturing
- Adaptable
- Energetic
- Analytical but decisive
- Sensitive to events

 Action point 2.5 – Enhancing your managerial effectiveness

A comprehensive range of aspects of clinical management have been discussed in this chapter. Based on areas such as the roles and qualities of an effective manager, reflect on the management component of your role, and identify how you will apply what you have learnt in this chapter to your everyday management practice together with your personal development needs.

You may find it helpful to compile an action plan, remembering that action plans include 'achieve by' dates, as well as identifying personnel and other resources that will help to achieve the objectives in the action plan. Therefore, reflect on the content of this chapter and identify your current managerial strengths and development needs using the format below. Some suggestions related to 'Human resource manager' are given as an example for guidance on how action plans could be constituted.

Managerial role development	Objectives	How will I achieve them & who can support me	Review and achieve by date
Human resource manager	Develop knowledge and competence in the performance of IDPRs	Attend in-house course for preparation as reviewer	Two months
		• Shadow my manager conducting an IDPR review • Discuss opportunities to conduct IDPRs for junior colleagues within the team • Complete a reflective account of an IDPR I complete	
Promoter of staff welfare			
Capacity manager			
Effectiveness and efficiency monitor			
Planner and communicator			
Decision-maker and problem-solver			
Quality assuror			
Guardian of health and safety			
Policy enforcer			
Staff trainer and educator			
Clinician and practice developer			
Leader and team worker			

It should be noted that objectives identified in action plans and personal development plans need to be SMART, that is, specific, measurable, achievable, realistic (or relevant) and timed. It also needs to be acknowledged that all management components identified above are underpinned by the necessary communication skills, with specific communication skill warranted by different situations, clinical specialisms and purposes, as discussed in Chapter 1.

Guidelines for effective management in practice settings

This chapter has examined theories and styles of management and the roles and personal qualities of clinical managers. The term effective is an adjective, which refers to being able to achieve or accomplish results. To 'effect' is to 'accomplish', and the noun 'effect' refers to 'something attained or acquired as the result of an action'. The closely related term 'efficient' also refers to being effective, but with the use of the least amount of effort and resources. Therefore, the effective and efficient DCM is one who achieves results of a pre-determined standard, and does so without waste of available human and non-human resources.

A number of strategies have been suggested to enable the DCM to reflect upon and self-assess their effectiveness as a manager. The managerial roles theory suggested in Figure 2.3 is one, Mintzberg's role theory is another, as is Fayol's (1949). Different guidelines for effective management practice are required, which comprise being proficient in the activities identified in Figure 2.3 as they are extracted from contemporary management practice. These guidelines are presented in Box 2.5.

Box 2.5: Guidelines for effective management practice – actions for success

- Work with people, and see your team members as your most valuable resources.
- Create appropriate mechanisms in order to enable employees to meet their social and psychological growth needs.
- Act as a role model, lead by example and endeavour to empathise with your staff.
- Take into account your employees' expectations of their employment, and what motivates them.
- Use an eclectic model that draws upon various theories to support how you manage.
- Ensure that each person feels important, and let them know that you appreciate them.
- Be accessible.
- Help individuals achieve their aspirations, as their success is reflected in yours.
- Distribute workload, responsibilities and new opportunities equitably.
- Treat people fairly but according to merit.

Chapter summary

It was noted early in this chapter that it is through the process of management that the activities of employees are co-ordinated and directed to ensure achievement of the healthcare organisation's goals. Management is consequently the launchpad and bedrock for organisational effectiveness, and is therefore concerned with appropriate utilisation of resources, human and non-human, in the provision of a service. The next chapter explores leadership theories and styles, a concept that is complementary to management.

This chapter has examined management theories roles and styles that should enable the DCM to manage practice settings effectively, and constituted discussions on:

- day-to-day activities of DCMs, their roles, styles and personal characteristics, as well as effective clinical management; a pragmatic approach in examining the extent to which existing knowledge on management can be applied to practice settings at the practical level, as well as taking an analytical stance;
- managing an area of the organisation, including managers and management, the structure of organisations and hierarchical levels within them;
- conventional management theories such as the classical approach, the human relations approach, the systems approach, the contingency approach and post-modern approaches as well as managerial role theory; it also examined management styles of healthcare managers;
- the qualities and personal skills of healthcare managers; and
- being an effective manager in the practice setting followed by management principles and guidelines.

THREE Leadership in practice settings

Introduction

Effective leadership is essential in healthcare services to drive care and treatment in the light of continuous policy changes and social expectations, some of which were discussed at the beginning of Chapter 1. As the lynchpin of care delivery, the DCM therefore needs to be equipped with appropriate leadership skills, which can be developed through leadership programmes. The chapter thus delves into the extensive literature on leadership and focuses on leadership skills that are most applicable in healthcare.

Chapter objectives

On completion of this chapter you will be able to:

- identify the reasons for studying leadership in healthcare;
- distinguish between the concepts leadership and management;
- demonstrate comprehensive knowledge of available theories and styles of leadership, and how the DCM can develop them;
- give an account of the ways in which power is a component of leadership, and the nature of power in practice settings; and
- cite some of the research studies on leadership, and some of the current leadership development programmes.

Why study leadership?

One of the reasons for examining leadership is that it comprises one of the essential roles of the manager as identified in the managerial role framework presented in Figure 2.3 in Chapter 2.

Action point 3.1 – Leaders and their attributes

Think of well-known leaders in healthcare in the following domains:

- Historical e.g. Florence Nightingale
- Within your own healthcare organisation
- An international leader

Now think about the attributes that they have that make them good leaders.

In response to the above action point, you might have felt that healthcare leaders as role models have to be first and foremost healthcare practitioners who inspire and lead by example, who actively engage in delivering patient care, and who are usually available to listen to suggestions for improving patient care and better ways of working. They might be more senior post-holders such as clinical managers, nurse (or allied health profession) consultants and practice educators. They would be healthcare practitioners who have the interests of their patients and their profession at heart.

Furthermore, Clegg (2000) notes that the satisfaction that staff achieve from their work is in part determined by the style of leadership they work under. Almio-Metcalf (1996) notes that leadership style and organisational culture are associated with an increase in productivity and staff satisfaction. In healthcare, there is a correlation between effective leadership and the quality of patient care and staff morale (Manley, 1997).

An organisation's success or failure is dependent upon its leaders, and all healthcare practitioners can be considered to be in positions where they can take the lead in some way. Furthermore, there does not seem to be any evidence that leadership qualities are inherited, or belong to one particular type of person. Research (e.g. Cunningham and Kitson, 2000; Kouzes and Posner, 2007) has indicated that leadership comprises competencies that can be learned through appropriate development programmes. The DCM, therefore, has the potential to be an effective leader within their practice setting.

The importance of leadership development has been emphasised in various policy publications including *The NHS Plan* (DH, 2000a), and *High Quality Care For All* (DH, 2008a) particularly as part of the NHS modernisation agenda. Various, leadership development programmes are offered by a number of providers to healthcare practitioners.

What is leadership?

Distinguishing between leadership and management

Action point 3.2 – Similarities and differences between leaders and managers

What are leaders and what do they do? Based on your own experiences of management and leadership in practice settings, consider the notions of being a manager and being a leader, and make notes on what you feel are the similarities and differences between these roles.

Various terms such as manager, leader, supervisor, head of the team, and even administrator are at times used interchangeably. In fact, management and leadership in particular are distinct entities albeit with overlapping functions.

The concept management and roles of managers were discussed in Chapter 2, indicating that management refers to activities and competencies of managers, while the term manager refers to the person who has been appointed to plan, organise, coordinate, supervise, negotiate, evaluate and integrate services with the use of resources made available to them by the organisation. Managers are given responsibility to ensure that the organisation's objectives are being achieved, and that all activities run smoothly. Managers need to exercise interpersonal skills and authority in this endeavour, and be accountable for their actions.

Leadership on the other hand is defined by Huczynski and Buchanan (2007:695) as 'the process of *influencing* the activities of an organised group in its efforts towards goal-setting and goal achievement'. Mullins (2007) sees leadership as a relationship through which one person *influences* the behaviour or actions of other people.

These are fairly standard definitions that indicate that leaders are individuals who exert influence and authority over others. In the context of the DCM's roles, leadership comprises the ability to motivate, inspire and energise individuals and groups to identify and achieve healthcare goals. To disentangle the term leadership further, it is important to note that leadership is a noun that can have four possible meanings, namely:

1   The activity of leading
2   The body of people who lead a group
3   The status of the leader
4   The ability to lead

It is also possible to distinguish between managers and leaders in that leadership is one of the roles of managers, as identified in Table 2.1 and Figure 2.3 in Chapter 2. Leadership is one of the managerial roles of DCMs, and is therefore a subset of management. The overall distinctions between leadership and management are that management is about monitoring and measuring performance against pre-determined goals, ensuring adherence to policies and procedures, maximising outputs and productivity, working within resource allocations, and controlling and organising necessary structures and systems. Leadership is about being visionary, showing the way forward, anticipating change, innovating, seeing the bigger picture, inspiring, motivating and focusing on the development of individuals.

The difference between management and leadership has also been explained by Watson's (1983) seven 'Ss' model which suggests that managers tend to rely on: strategy, structure and systems, whereas leaders utilise the soft Ss, namely: style, staff, skills and shared goals.

Leadership is thus a dynamic two-way process based on a leader–follower relationship. McGregor (1987) suggests that leadership is a dynamic form of behaviour with a number of variables affecting the leadership relationship, namely:

• Characteristics of the leader,
• Attitude, needs and other personal characteristics of the followers,
• Nature of the organisation, such as its purpose, its structure, the tasks to be performed, and
• Social, economic and political environment.

Hollingsworth (1999) suggests that managers can learn leadership development from the armed forces. He suggests that there are six fundamental differences between managers and leaders:

1   Managers administer – leaders innovate
2   Managers maintain – leaders develop
3   Managers focus on systems and structure – leaders focus on people
4   Managers rely on control – leaders inspire trust
5   Managers keep an eye on the bottom line – leaders have an eye on the horizon
6   Managers do things right – leaders do the right thing.

Robinson (1999) and others disagree with Hollingsworth, suggesting that the above list may be accepted if the term manager is replaced by 'administrator'. However, these suggestions indicate that managers are more concerned with ensuring that the organisation functions smoothly, and achieving organisational or departmental aims, whereas the leader is more people oriented. Being staff-oriented and having shared goals is clearly more people-oriented management.

Furthermore, Gratton (2000) suggests that the very nature of management methods is currently changing, and has moved away from an emphasis on getting results by close control of the workforce towards an environment of coaching, support and empowerment, that is leading. Leaders are accountable for their followers' performance, which they achieve by helping them to be efficient, and to develop their strengths and abilities (Murphy, 2005).

Whose leadership?

In addition to the concept that managers have a leadership role, there are also ways of distinguishing between different types of leaders. The key ones are delineated in Box 3.1.

Box 3.1: Different types of leadership

Traditional leadership	When authority or power rests on an established belief in the sanctity of traditional and historical leaders such as a prince. Family traditions and social ties directly influence the continuity of this form of leadership.
Formal leadership	Practised by the individual with *legitimate authority* conferred by the organisation and described as an aspect of the approved position. This could be a *formally* appointed clinical manager or a project leader for instance. It is also referred to as legal/rational leader.

Box 3.1: Continued

Informal leadership	Is exercised by a staff member who does not have a specified management role, but has *knowledge, personal status and skills* in persuading and guiding others.
Attempted leadership	Where an individual in a group attempts to exert influence over other members of the group.
Successful or effective leadership	Brings about the behaviour and results that were intended by the leader, and in the achievement of group goals.
Naturally emerging or charismatic leadership	Lead through natural charm.
Shared leadership	Such as when two or more band 6 RNs share leadership in a practice setting because they are of equal status.
Elected leadership	For example the prime minister.
Imposed leadership	For instance on appointment as a manager, the individual also adopts a leadership role.

All clinicians should be able to easily identify various types of leadership in different practice settings. For instance, in the context of nursing, the notion of shared leadership can be found in teams with several employees on the same pay bands such as in a community mental health team. However, a leader is not a leader unless they have followers, and people who provide support.

 Action point 3.3 – Leader and follower

Think of aspects of your work in which you are a leader, and aspects in which you are a follower. Consider the ways in which your approaches to your work vary as these different roles change.

Theories and styles of leadership

Several theories of leadership have emerged over the years endeavouring to disentangle the concept and its practical applications. As suggested in Chapter 2, a theory implies that if a certain action is taken in a particular way, then a certain predictable effect can be expected.

Action point 3.4 – Effective leadership

Prior to delving into established theories of leadership, consider the following, and the significance for healthcare. Think of a senior healthcare practitioner in your organisation who is a good leader, and decide what it is about them that makes them a good leader. Contrast this to someone who you consider to be a poor leader. Complete columns A and B as illustrated below:

Column A: *An effective leader is*	Column B: *An ineffective leader*
• An effective communicator • Approachable …	• Does not share information effectively • Inaccessible and is unapproachable …

The purpose of Action point 3.4 was to sensitise you to published theories of leadership. Over the years, leadership theorists have viewed the subject from different perspectives and four prominent groups of theories can be identified (see Box 3.2). Wisely, contemporary leadership theories do not discard previous theories, although some theories are still at experimental stages, and might not have gained wide acceptance within social sciences yet.

Box 3.2: Prominent leadership theories

There are four main groups of leadership theories:

1 *Trait approach*
   • Characteristics of leaders

2 *Functional approach*
   • Action-centred leadership

3 *Behavioural and style theories*
   • Leadership styles
   • The managerial grid

4 *Contemporary theories*
   • Charismatic leader
   • Connective leadership
   • Servant leadership
   • Transactional leadership
   • Transformational leadership

The chapter will now focus on analysing these competing theories.

Trait theories

By the 1950s hundreds of studies had already been conducted exploring the specific characteristics of effective leaders (Handy, 1993). These studies were aimed at ascertaining the characteristics of people who are leaders, differentiating them from non-leaders. Trait theories, also known as 'great man' or 'great woman' theories, of leadership attempt to identify inborn traits of successful leaders. Subsequent studies elicited significant correlation between leadership effectiveness and the following traits:

- Intelligence
- Supervisory ability
- Initiative
- Self-assurance
- Individuality

Based on several research studies Bass (1990) developed a profile of traits that are evident in successful leaders. These are categorised in three areas as:

- *Intelligence*
  - Judgement
  - Decisiveness
  - Knowledge
  - Fluency
- *Personality*
  - Adaptability
  - Alertness
  - Integrity
  - Nonconformity
- *Ability*
  - Cooperativeness
  - Popularity
  - Tact

The trait approach has both its proponents and its critics. The key problems with trait theories are that:

- traits are difficult to define accurately or understand fully;
- there are many exceptional leaders who do not possess all identified leadership traits;
- possession of most or few of these traits does not mean that a person is a better or worse manager or leader; and
- it is questionable whether an individual could have all the traits.

Another difficulty with the trait approach is that if individual traits or characteristics are seen to be responsible for effective functioning as leaders, then the question arises whether people are born with these traits or characteristics, or whether they have learned them, through either self-teaching or through attending courses.

However trait theories have not been completely disregarded despite several other leadership theories having emerged over the years. For instance, Wright (1996) suggests that some leadership traits can be ascribed as unique to nursing leadership positions, such as being a clinical expert, a change agent, an ordinary person and a centred human being who uses 'head and heart'. Based on ongoing research, Kouzes and Posner (2007) conclude that 'Admired Leaders' tend to elicit specific characteristics, whereupon 50 per cent or more respondents selected:

- Honest (88%)
- Forward looking (71%)
- Competent (66%)
- Inspiring (65%)

As many as 28 to 47 per cent of respondents selected intelligent, fair-minded, broad-minded, supportive, straightforward, dependable, co-operative, determined and imaginative as specific characteristics of effective leaders; less than 25 per cent of respondents selected ambitious, courageous, caring, mature, loyal, self-controlled and independent. However, there is no complete agreement on the nature and essential characteristics of a leader, nor on what an effective leader is. It can be seen as an attribute of position, or of knowledge or wisdom; it can be based on personality functions or in terms of the ability to achieve effective work performance by followers.

Furthermore, the Myers Briggs Personality Types (Teamtechnology, 2008) provides a widely used typology for identifying the personality of individuals aspiring to team leadership positions. It comprises assessment of the individual on four spectrums, namely: extraversion and introversion, sensing and intuition, thinking and feeling and judging and perceiving, which are dimensions that can be used as self-assessment and subsequent development of these qualities.

The functional approach

The functional (or group) approach to leadership focuses on the functions of the leader, and thereby also bypasses the overlapping concepts of appointed versus naturally emerging leader. It indicates that in either case the leader can learn to elicit the right functions at the right time. Kotter (1990) suggests that by concentrating on the functions of the leader, their performance can be improved by training and thus leadership skills can be learnt, developed and perfected. Kotter (1990) also indicates that organisations should not wait for leaders to come along, but 'grow' their own by identifying employees with potential. This approach therefore also supports the notion that several members of a professional group can have scope to develop their leadership potential and exercise leadership skills.

Adair's action-centred leadership

A more current function-related leadership theory is Adair's (2005) action-centred leadership (ACL), according to which, the leader functions by paying attention to three sets of needs: task needs, individual needs and team maintenance needs. The effectiveness of the leader is dependent upon meeting these three areas of need within the work group. Too much concern for any one of these three areas can cause imbalance, and can interfere with the productiveness and effectiveness of the group. This could consequently affect the quality of the outcomes, the morale of the group, its motivation and accomplishment.

In healthcare organisations, leaders need to pay attention to all three sets of needs, immaterial of whether the leadership position is attained through appointment, or through natural emergence.

 Action point 3.5 – Applying ACL

Consider the DCM's activities as the clinical leader from Adair's action-centred leadership viewpoint. Then, make notes on how the DCM can endeavour to meet the needs of those who are led effectively within your practice setting, categorising their actions under task, individual and team needs.

The DCM can utilise Adair's (2005) action-centred leadership in various ways. For meeting task needs, they can ensure that objectives of the work group are achieved, resources are allocated as appropriate and they delegate according to capabilities. For meeting team or group needs, they can hold appropriate team meetings, make themselves approachable and available and give feedback. For meeting individual needs, they can conduct IDPRs regularly, and be aware of any conflict and potential problem areas in interpersonal relationships within the team.

To ensure leadership effectiveness, all three sets of needs, task, group and individual have to be met. It may appear that some items in a particular column could well correspond with another column, but this is immaterial, as the main purpose of ACL is to ensure an integrated approach to one's leadership functions.

Behavioural theories and styles of leadership

Leadership behaviours have been classified in several different ways. Some of the more widely accepted ones include traditional leadership styles and the managerial grid style.

Traditional leadership styles

There are many ways of categorising leadership styles, the traditional classification being authoritarian (or autocratic), democratic (or participative), permissive (or laissez-faire) and bureaucratic.

- *Authoritarian*
  - Focuses on power and need for authority and approval of status by others
  - Exercises control and directive behaviour
  - Makes decisions alone and expects obedience of instructions
  - Uses undertones of coercion.
- *Democratic*
  - Formally seeks the views of all relevant parties

- – Displays a wish to consult and work with individuals and teams
- – Uses the human relations approach
- – Engages in open two-way communication
- – Encourages collaborative teamwork
- *Permissive*
  - – Uses few established rules and policies
  - – Monitors performance from a distance, and therefore might appear detached
  - – Permits individual and teams to work autonomously
- *Bureaucratic*
  - – Follows established policies and rules to the letter
  - – Power is exercised by applying fixed and inflexible rules
  - – Communications are impersonal
  - – Only makes new decisions based on norms

Despite the approving and disapproving overtones of each of these styles of leadership, it is useful to ascertain more clearly what the likely merits or weaknesses of each style might be.

Action point 3.6 – Merits and drawbacks of different styles of leadership

Based on your experience of professional leadership, consider the effects, that is, the strengths and weaknesses of each of the following styles of leadership.

- Autocratic
- Participative
- Laissez-faire
- Bureaucratic

Now consider clinical situations when the various styles identified appear more appropriate.

Many of the positive effects and drawbacks of each style were identified just before this action point. Leadership styles can also vary according to specific clinical circumstances. For example, in a situation where an unexpected violent episode occurs in a mental health practice setting, or a team of paramedics dealing with an emergency situation, the leadership style may be more directive (or authoritarian). In situations where there is no immediate risk to individual safety, more democratic styles may be adopted. Other leadership styles can be considered such as those identified in Box 3.1, including political leadership.

The managerial grid style of leadership

Blake and McCanse (1991) note that there are four identifiable leadership styles that can be plotted in a two-dimensional grid, as discussed in Chapter 2 as a style of management. Leadership style refers to the way in which the leader carries out their functions, that is, the way in which the leader is perceived as typically behaving towards their followers. Such leaders are developed through education, training and life experiences, assuming that effective leaders acquire a pattern (or style) of learned behaviours. Therefore style refers to how as leaders we behave on a day-to-day basis, because we know or have learnt from previous experience that the way we do things works.

Contemporary leadership theories

In addition to trait, functional and behavioural theories of leadership, the more current approaches are referred to as contemporary theories. To an extent however, contemporary theories represent further development of the earlier leadership theories, and take into account current social, political and organisational factors. Some of the more prominent contemporary leadership theories are:

- Charismatic
- Connective
- Servant
- Transactional
- Transformational

Charismatic leadership Charm, persuasiveness, personal power, self-confidence, extraordinary ideas and strong (often unconventional) convictions are the main personal qualities that characterise charismatic leaders. The leader's personality arouses affection and emotional commitment, first to the leader, and second to the beliefs and causes the leader espouses. However, charisma as an individual quality is difficult to define and has not been scientifically tested adequately, and the theory goes against the current belief that leadership skills can be developed or learned (DH, 2000c).

Connective leadership As a theory that recognises the role of leaders as fostering collaborative intra-organisational and inter-organisational relationships, Klakovich (1994) suggests that connective leadership provides either a separate or supplementary theory to contemporary clinical leadership. This theory suggests that the activities of contemporary leaders must include the ability to create inter-connections between and across practice settings, the purpose of which is to better coordinate and integrate patient care services in a caring, non-competitive, collegial manner.

Charns and Tewksbury (1993) explain that the process of creating connections and fostering integration requires that the leader:

i   identifies actual and potential collaborators;
ii   communicates and sells a potential shared vision to those in varied settings and in disparate conditions;
iii   describes the value each collaborator could bring to the endeavour both to the individual and others;
iv   facilitates communication by sharing information, preparing for interactions and follow-up on communication exchanges;
v   builds and maintains social interactions and comfort;
vi   defines and sells roles and assignments;

vii   tracks and rewards contributions;
viii   formalises an integrated effort at the right time.

However, this theory seems limited, as being well connected through networking is already a recognised essential attribute of most effective leaders in current day healthcare.

Servant leadership   As another distinct leadership theory, servant leadership comprises being a leader primarily because of the wish to do good for one's followers (e.g. Greenleaf, 1991). It therefore entails taking an altruistic stance, and is based on the premise that leadership originates from a desire to serve, and not so much because one's job role includes being a leader, or other reasons. It could be argued that politicians take on servant leadership roles because they choose to serve the public.

Howatson-Jones (2004) commends the use of servant leadership theory in healthcare, noting that this approach incorporates the leader endeavouring to ascertain 'the followers' perspectives as a better way to promote effectiveness. The servant leader can lead healthcare practitioners by empathising with them, considering their job role, views and aspirations. Servant leadership is therefore about serving the needs of the followers and empowering them, and thereby includes a stewardship element. The likely weakness with the servant leadership approach is that if the organisation's needs are considered as secondary, then the amount of work done, that is, productivity, could suffer.

Transactional leadership   Based on the presumption that one doesn't have to be a natural leader to manage, nor a manager to lead, transactional leadership theory relates to leading by virtue of the management position held in the organisational hierarchy. This approach is closely related to the achievement of organisational goals, which in healthcare trusts constitutes attending to the health of the local population. Transactional leadership is founded on the theory that leaders are successful or effective to the extent that they aim to maintain equilibrium and harmony by fulfilling their roles according to policies and procedures and use incentives to enhance employee loyalty and performance (Bass and Riggio, 2006).

Although this approach supports and maintains the status quo, and has firm elements of predictability, it has also been criticised for lacking vision for the future of organisations and healthcare in general.

Transformational leadership theory   Transformational leadership is a widely advocated leadership approach for healthcare. It entails aspiring to effect revolutionary changes (Bass and Riggio, 2006; Kouzes and Posner, 2007), and focuses on merging the goals, desires and values of leaders and followers into a common goal. It refers to 'the ability of leaders to influence others by transforming their behaviour without necessarily being in a position of authority' (Morgan, 2005:27). The objective of this is to generate employees' commitment to the organisation's vision and ideal, in conjunction with their own individual aspirations and aims for the organisation.

Murphy (2005) suggests that transformational leaders are visionary, balanced, self-aware and confident in breaking professional boundaries to develop a multidisciplinary team approach to patient care. Using transformational leadership, the leader appeals to individuals' 'better selves', and fosters followers' innate wishes to pursue higher values. Transformational leaders encourage others to exercise leadership, and inspire followers by instilling a belief that the followers have the ability to achieve exceptional aims. It depends on the leader's ability to stimulate growth and development, and to discourage dependence. Consequently, the transformational leader is 'the catalyst for creating new innovative organisational paradigms' (Murphy, 2005:135).

While acknowledging that the key elements of leadership are leaders' personal characteristics, their interpersonal relationships, teamwork and being role models, it can be deduced from the above-mentioned points that the transformational model of leadership is most appropriate for healthcare, and without it practice improvement is less likely to occur.

The transformational leadership style is described by Markham (1998) as collaborative, consultative and consensus seeking, and as ascribing power to interpersonal skills and personal contact. Kouzes and Posner (2007) identify five key practices in transformational leadership:

1 Challenging the process
2 Inspiring shared vision
3 Enabling others to act
4 Modelling the way
5 Encouraging the heart.

 Action point 3.7 – The vision in transformational leadership

The term transformational implies being visionary, that is, having ideas and aspirations of how things could be different for the better (Murphy, 2005), and then implementing those visions. Such concepts directly apply to all healthcare practitioners and practice settings in the quest for continually raising standards of care and treatment. What is your vision of how care can be delivered, organised or led better in your own practice setting, and in your healthcare organisation?

An organisation's vision for its future can be contrasted with Blake and McCanse's (1991) styles of leadership which explore the effects of 'concern for people' and 'concern for production', the latter focusing on patient care. This was discussed in Chapter 2. A comparison of a leader who utilises the transformational approach to one who uses transactional theory of leadership is presented on Table 3.1.

The two approaches are therefore different in that while transactional leadership is predominantly concerned about managerial 'transactions' between the manager and the managed, transformational leadership constitutes endeavouring to make more radical changes that can present challenges and growth for all. Transactional leadership constitutes orderly breaking down of tasks although this can often be limited in vision

Table 3.1 *Comparison of transformational and transactional leadership approaches*

Transformational leadership	Transactional leadership
• Merges own and followers' goals, desires and values and that of the organisations into a common goal	• Aims to maintain equilibrium and status quo
• Generates employee commitment to the vision	• Is task-centred and orderly
• Inspires and instils a belief in followers that they have the ability to do exceptional things	• Performs tasks strictly according to policies and procedures
• Stimulates growth and development by discouraging dependence	• Has a short- or medium-term focus
• Challenges subordinates	• Coaches and fosters sheltered learning
• Rewards informally and personally	• Uses extrinsic rewards
• Is emotional, passionate about existing and new ventures	• High self-interest
• Sees home and work on a continuum	• Sees home and work as separate entities

and energy. Transformational leadership constitutes keeping a strategic or helicopter view of the whole.

The five contemporary theories of leadership relate to existing knowledge on leadership, but for more useful implementation, further research through structured empirical studies will be needed to firm up their application potential in different settings.

Leadership and power

Most definitions of leadership incorporate the 'influence' of the leader over those who they lead. Leadership influence is dependent upon the type of power that the leader exercises over those who they lead. Power can be defined as the capacity to produce or prevent a specific change. Various types of power can be identified, as illustrated in Box 3.3.

Box 3.3: Types of power

PERSONAL POWER
Expert (or profession) power Based on the profession or occupation of the individual, together with possession of the unique knowledge, skills and expertise associated with their role; seen as competent; usually limited to narrow well-defined specialism

---

Box 3.3: Continued

Referent (or ascribed/status) power	Based on the perceptions of others, admiration and respect for an individual, and identification with the leader; the leader with perceived reputation, charisma and attractiveness; position in society i.e. wealth
Connection power	Based on the individual's formal and informal links to influential or prestigious persons within and outside an area or organisation

ORGANISATIONAL POWER

Reward power	Based on inducements such as pay, promotion, praise and recognition that the leader can offer group members in exchange for co-operation and contributions that advance the group's objectives
Punishment or coercive power	Based on penalties a leader has ability to impose on an individual or a group such as withdrawal of support, invoking disciplinary procedures and withholding promotion
Authority or legitimate power	Based on the position (or job and rank) that the individual holds within the hierarchy of the organisation; stems from the leader's right to make a request because of the authority in an organisational hierarchy – not so much on personal relationships
Information power	Based on access to valued data

 Action point 3.8 – Power

Taking into account all of the healthcare practitioners who have input into care delivery in your practice setting, try and identify individuals who actually exercise power of one or another of the seven types of power identified in Box 3.3.

Leaders are individuals who stand out from others in the degree of influence that they have on their thinking, motivation and activities. In response to Action point 3.8, you are likely to have identified individuals who have one or more forms of power detailed in Box 3.3. As a minimum the DCM has legitimate power, and possibly other elements such as, referent power.

Guidelines for the effective use of these different forms of power in organisations suggested by Yukl (2002) are presented in Table 3.2.

Similar guidelines can be constituted for the other types of power identified in Box 3.3.

Table 3.2 *Guidelines for effective use of two types of power in organisations*

i) **Using legitimate authority or power (organisational power)**	ii) **Using reward power (personal power)**
• Use politeness and clarity when making requests • Explain the reasons for requests • Do not exceed your scope of authority • Verify authority if necessary • Follow agreed organisational channels • Follow up to ascertain compliance • Insist on compliance if necessary	• Offer the type of rewards that people desire • Ensure rewards are fair and ethical • Do not make promises of more than you can deliver • Identify and publish simple criteria for giving rewards • Provide rewards as promised when requirements have been met • Use rewards symbolically (not in a manipulative way).

Research on clinical leadership

A fair range of research has been published on clinical leadership. Earlier research on leadership has tended to be directed at particular aspects of leadership such as:

- Leadership attributes/skills
- Leadership traits (not attributes)
- Style and effect of leadership
- Effective leadership.

With a laissez-faire approach the least work gets done. More recently, on exploring leadership effectiveness, Goleman (2000) concluded that the most effective leaders tend to combine different leadership styles for different situations, as they consider appropriate. However, there are several variables that can affect the effectiveness of the leader in the workplace. These variables include a range of aspects of management such as availability of resources, namely, equipment and materials, the relationship between the manager and employees, and external influences such as legislation and pressure groups.

Specific to practice settings, Cook (2001) used the grounded theory approach to explore the concept of effective leadership of clinical nurse leaders which he suggested also applies to leaders in other healthcare professions. The five key attributes of effective leaders and associated 'facilitative factors' are as follows:

1 *Highlighting*
   - Freedom to act
   - Willingness to negotiate
   - Questioning attitude encouraged

- Willing to learn from others
- Clinical expertise and knowledge

2 *Respecting*
- Empathy and understanding
- Self-motivation
- Being valued
- Concern for staff

3 *Influencing*
- Organising others with forethought
- Assessing ability on delegation
- Motivating others
- Instilling confidence
- Proving oneself in the field of practice

4 *Creativity*
- Ability to prioritise
- Planning ahead
- Maintaining an overview
- Aiding information flow

5 *Supporting*
- Facilitated to organise self and own workload
- Time for planning
- Empowered to adapt the working environment to improve practice
- Moving purposefully

Clegg (2000) reports on a study on the successful application of transformational leadership on team performance and the quality of patient care in a community trust, the results of which are said to be encouraging as they could clearly demonstrate an improvement in the quality of the care they deliver as a result of their quest for excellence. Lipley (2004) reports on an extensive study conducted by the University of Sheffield that suggests that a mix of transformational leadership and transactional leadership is better than the laissez-faire approach at making staff more enthusiastic about their jobs.

Opinion literature and published research on leadership in healthcare abounds, and new research in the field will no doubt appear in the future. However, many of these studies are on leadership related largely to key initiatives or projects on the management of specific medical conditions or health education, not to researching leadership as a concept in its own right.

Current leadership initiatives and skills development programmes

Policy documents by the DH (2000c) and the general literature on clinical leadership suggest that all healthcare professionals may be in positions where they take the lead in some way, and can be leaders in different components of healthcare provision, and at different levels in the management hierarchy.

For actual leadership skill development, individuals might need to attend appropriate courses or workshops, based on self-assessment of knowledge and skills, and identifying self-development areas to work on. Various leadership development programmes are available. The development of the titles 'clinical leader' and 'team leader' have emerged, both comprising leaders at the practice edge of healthcare. However, one of the more prominent nursing leadership development courses has been the Royal College of Nursing's (RCN, 2005a) Clinical Leadership Programme (CLP).

Existing knowledge of leadership needs to be built on by application of theories to current healthcare contexts. It is advocated by many though that team leaders need ongoing development programmes, together with the managerial support to fulfil these roles (Anon, 1998; Binnie, 1998). Healthcare practitioners are being encouraged to become lifelong learners, a concept that has fast become a substantive and unavoidable component of healthcare provision (Gopee, 2001), and a core skill for clinical leadership development.

The preferred leadership theory base adopted by many development programmes is primarily transformational leadership, as it challenges autocratic unilateral leadership approaches, and because other leadership theories implicate inborn leadership qualities. Transformational leadership is also preferred to transactional leadership theory as the latter tends to be related to management functions, which is to 'get the day-to-day job done', and could imply 'imposed leadership' (Cook, 2001). An extensive range of qualities and abilities are cited in leadership literature on effective transformational leadership. Those identified by Murphy (2005) are:

- Being a visionary
- Being a futurist
- Being a catalyst for change
- Exercising persuasive and captivating communication
- Stimulating fervent emotions
- Influencing beliefs, attitudes and behaviours
- Promoting motivation and commitment through interpersonal communication
- Displaying honesty, integrity, commitment and credibility
- Encouraging staff to become independent, responsible, and autonomous in their decision-making
- Possessing high self-esteem, self-regard and self-awareness.

Several leadership self-assessment and skill development tools are available in textbooks (e.g. Marriner Tomey 2004; Kouzes and Posner, 2007); journals articles (e.g. McNichol and Smith, 2001; Murphy, 2005); and via the Internet. McNichol and Smith (2001) for instance report on a Leadership Effectiveness Analysis (LEA) psychometrically validated instrument, which constitutes 22 leadership behaviours as 128 statements that can form the basis for self-assessment of strengths and developmental needs. Subsequently, appropriate learning actions can be taken.

Guidelines for effective clinical leadership

A number of leadership theories, styles, competences and attributes have been examined in this chapter, including Murphy (2005) and Cook and Leathard (2004). It can be concluded that ultimately it is the specific skills or the performance and leadership styles displayed and exercised by healthcare practitioners in clinical leadership positions that determine their effectiveness.

Action point 3.9 – Effective leadership

Various activities undertaken through this chapter will have facilitated greater insight into leadership traits, functions, styles and theories. For this final action point, focus on the characteristics of effective leaders. Draw 3 columns and 12 rows on a sheet of paper as illustrated in Table 3.3, and record Kouzes and Posner's (2007) practices of 'Exemplary Leaders' in the left-hand column, which are to:

- be more effective in meeting job-related demands;
- be more successful in representing their units to upper management;
- create higher-performing teams;
- foster renewed loyalty and commitment;
- increase motivational levels and willingness to work hard;
- promote higher levels of involvement in schools;
- enlarge the size of their congregations;
- raise more money and expand gift-giving levels;
- extend the range of their agency's services;
- reduce absenteeism, turnover and dropout rates; and
- possess high degrees of personal credibility.

These practices also comprise a comprehensive range of skills of an effective clinical leader. Perform a self-assessment on these 'practices' making notes in the second and third columns on how you see yourself as a leader now, and your aspirations as a leader, respectively.

Table 3.3 *Construing leadership*

Characteristics of an effective leader	Me as I am now	My ideal self as a clinical leader

Amongst others, both the qualities and abilities of effective transformational leaders identified by Murphy (2005), and the practices of 'Exemplary Leaders' identified by Kouzes and Posner's (2007) comprise best practice guidelines for clinical leadership'.

Table 3.3 can clearly be utilised to identify areas of self-development as a clinical leader. When you have completed these columns, you may choose to discuss them with colleagues of senior, junior and equal status, to obtain external views of your abilities and development plans, a concept and exercise referred to as 360 degree feedback (Faugier and Woolnough, 2003; Kouzes and Posner, 2007). With 360 degree feedback, it is essential that a supportive medium is created, possibly by utilising an external facilitator so that the receiver of the feedback does not feel over-criticised.

Chapter summary

Healthcare practice comprises providing leadership to individuals and teams of healthcare practitioners as an inherent component of the management of care. A number of clinical leadership development programmes have emerged mainly because of limited evidence of leadership activities and role models at the close of the last century. They are largely based on piloted projects, and opportunities are more widely available to healthcare practitioners with the ultimate view being to achieve consistency in the highest quality of care within the NHS. In this context, this chapter has explored:

- the reasons for requiring effective leadership in healthcare delivery and provision;
- definitions and the exact nature of leadership, that is, what it is, types of leadership, and ways in which leadership and management are different but overlapping concepts and activities;
- the various theories and styles of leadership that can be applied to lead effectively in healthcare, including trait theories, the functional approach such as action-centred leadership, behavioural theories and styles of leadership namely leadership styles, the managerial grid style of leadership and contingency styles of leadership;
- the significance of different types of power as an aspect of leadership, and guidelines for effective use of power in organisations; and
- research on leadership, and a number of recent and current initiatives and programmes on clinical leadership skill development.

FOUR Decision-making and problem-solving in practice settings

Introduction

The theories, principles and practice of management and leadership in healthcare were examined in Chapters 2 and 3. Both functions involve healthcare practitioners and DCMs making several decisions and resolving issues during the course of their day-to-day work. In recognition of these crucial management activities, this chapter focuses on the concepts decision-making and problem-solving.

Incorporated in this analysis are the theoretical knowledge, skills and systematic approaches to decision-making and problem-solving that the DCM can draw on, as well as the use of personal and professional experience and intuition. Conflict can be a feature of clinical management, and therefore how conflict is managed and resolved is also explored.

Chapter objectives

On completion of this chapter you will be able to:

- identify a wide range of decisions made by healthcare practitioners and analyse the significance of these decisions;
- explain the exact nature of, and distinctions between, the terms decision-making and problem-solving;
- explain the basis on which healthcare decisions are made, and the systematic approaches that can be used in both making decisions and solving problems in practice settings;
- enunciate the nature of conflict and how conflict in practice settings can be managed and resolved successfully; and
- feel prepared to engage in opportunities to practise professional decision-making and problem-solving skills.

Day-to-day personal and professional decisions and their significance

Day-to-day decision-making

 Action point 4.1 – Day-to-day decisions

a) Consider the actual decisions that you make in both your personal and professional life, and compile a list of:

- personal decisions made from the point that you woke up this morning, such as, what clothes to wear; and
- decisions made over the course of a particular span of duty (professional decisions), such as, what tasks to delegate to which member of staff.

Allow 5 to 10 minutes for this part of the action point and note these instances of decisions on a plain sheet of paper leaving a 5-centimetre margin on the right hand side of the paper for parts (b) and (c).

b) Consider which of these decisions were made consciously, and which were made subconsciously.

c) Now decide which of these decisions were in fact problems being solved, and write PS against them; and write DM against those that were not problems being solved.

On reviewing the items in the list, you will appreciate that we make numerous decisions, small and big, during the course of time, minute-by-minute, and day-by-day. Some of the professional and personal decisions identified by healthcare practitioners studying on management modules are listed in Table 4.1.

Table 4.1 *Personal and professional decisions*

Personal decisions made so far today	Professional decisions made over a particular shift or two
What to wear	What patient to allocate to which staff
What to have for breakfast, what cereals to eat	Whether to discharge a patient
Whether to put the washing out	Whether to apply for the new post/job
How to spend lunch break	What to tell a relative regarding the condition of a patient
What to cook for tea	
Whether to call course peer	What dressing to use
Whether to telephone teacher regarding daughter	Whether to go to a meeting on a new care package
Whether to reset snooze/sleep button	
Whether to have another cup of coffee	Ensuring the next shift is covered
How to get son to swimming lessons at 4 p.m.	Whether to give more time to a particular patient

One of the aims of Action point 4.1 was to start to distinguish between the activities that involve decision-making and those that involve problem-solving, as they are different concepts (see Box 4.1).

Box 4.1: Is it decision-making or is it problem-solving?

What to have for breakfast/what cereals to eat	Decision-making
How to get son to swimming lessons at 4 p.m.	Problem-solving
Walk to work or go by car	Decision-making
Whether to put the washing out	Decision-making
Whether to attend a lecture	Decision-making
Whether to call on course peer	Problem-solving
Whether to apply for the new post/job	Decision-making
Which patient to allocate to which staff	Decision-making or problem-solving
Which patients to visit (Community)	Decision-making
Whether to discharge a patient	Decision-making
Whether to give more time to a patient	Decision-making
Which dressing to use	Decision-making
Whether the next shift is covered	Problem-solving
Which staff to send on a transfer	Decision-making
What to tell a patient regarding the condition of their ill baby	Problem-solving

---

You will have noted no doubt that some of the activities listed in Box 4.1, such as what patient to allocate to which staff, can entail either a decision being made and a problem being solved, or both simultaneously.

Decision-making and problem-solving as important DCM functions

The DCM's role as decision maker and problem solver is one of the 12 managerial roles in clinical management identified in Chapter 2 (Figure 2.3). Previously, Mintzberg (1990) identified ten key roles of managers, four of which, that is, entrepreneur, disturbance handler, resource allocator and negotiator are grouped as 'decisional roles'.

Decision-making in relation to care delivery is a function of all healthcare practitioners involved in patient care by sheer virtue of their contract of employment and their professional body's code of professional practice. For the more junior healthcare practitioner, the decision might be when to report a patient observation to the doctor, for instance; and for a more senior healthcare practitioner this may involve deciding at which point to increase the dose of a particular medication.

What is decision-making and what is problem-solving?

Definitions and distinctions

So what is decision-making and what is problem-solving, and what if any are the similarities and differences between them? As noted in Action point 4.1, some decisions are clearly decisions being made and not problems being solved. Other situations are clearly problems being solved. Additionally, a decision being made can entail taking action to prevent a potential problem occurring.

For instance, ensuring safe staff:patient ratios when a colleague telephones in sick is a problem being solved. This can be done by reviewing the workload and patient dependency to establish if cover is required, and asking a team member to do a split shift or borrowing a staff member from another practice setting. In another instance, the DCM could be invited to attend a meeting to discuss a new record keeping system. This would be a decision that they have to make as by attending the meeting they would contribute towards the design of new documentation on the one hand, but on the other they are also being taken away from patient care delivery.

Consequently, decision-making entails considering several components of the situation and ultimately selecting one specific course of action. However, a straight forward act as it might sound, decision-making often comprises making a number of smaller but crucial sub-decisions. It requires accessing and collecting appropriate facts which lead to the final action. An open mind is often needed which allows a total view of the situation to be gained. It is also important to consider the availability of evidence, previous experience and the use of professional judgement.

The notion of problem-solving is different in that there is clearly a problem involved or that something is about to go wrong, and that some action needs to be taken to resolve or avert it. Indeed, dictionaries define the word problem as 'a doubtful or difficult matter, or a seemingly insoluble quandary' (Brown, 2002:2353). A decision-making situation does not always include a problem. Nonetheless, the two notions tend to be treated jointly and even used interchangeably. Problem-solving usually requires making decisions, and as became apparent in Action point 4.1, some activities encompass both notions. However, there are distinctions between the two terms as illustrated in Box 4.2.

Micro- and macro-decisions

Decisions, like problems, can be small or big. That is some decisions are straightforward and simple in that very few variables are involved, while others are more complex as many more variables have to be considered in reaching the decision. Nonetheless, most healthcare decisions involve a number of smaller or micro-decisions. For instance, consider how many sub-decisions the healthcare practitioner has to make when administering an intravenous bolus of antibiotics? Box 4.3, although not an exhaustive list, identifies a number of these micro-decisions, which are akin to reflection-in-action (Boud et al., 1985), and which involves continuous thinking about every single action being taken, in conjunction with justifiable rationales for them, and any associated evidence base.

Box 4.2: Distinctions between decision-making and problem-solving

Problem-solving

- Involves diagnosing a problem and solving it through a set of decisions

- May entail one or more correct solutions

Decision-making

- May not involve a problem, as a number of decisions are made routinely without seeing them as problems

- Always involves selecting one specific decision and related actions

- Often decision-making is a subset of problem-solving i.e. decisions are made on how to solve or avert the problem

Box 4.3: Micro decisions and reflection-in-action when administering intravenous bolus antibiotics

Am I competent to administer this IV drug? – No >
    Yes
    ↓
Do I know why is it being given? e.g. wound infection – No >
    Yes
    ↓
Is it prescribed correctly? – No >
    Yes
    ↓
Is the medication in stock? – No >
    Yes
    ↓
Expiry date checked? – No >
    Yes
    ↓
Draw prescribed amount in correct syringe, tray, etc.
    Yes
    ↓
Check correct patient, drug, dosage, route, time, ... – No >
    Yes
    ↓
Patient's consent/permission – No >
    Yes
    ↓

Box 4.3: Continued

Access site healthy? – No >
                    Yes
                     ↓
Administer over x minutes
                     ↓
What conversation should I engage patient in?
                     ↓
State of surrounding tissue when administering
                     ↓
Patient reaction? – OK
                     ↓
etc.

Similar sets of micro-decisions are made in other areas of healthcare, whether it involves enabling an agitated youngster in an Adolescent Unit to relax; enabling a woman with a complicated pregnancy to give birth safely; supporting a suicidal patient to avoid self-harm; or a practice nurse helping a group of patients to give up smoking. Many of these micro-decisions are made in seconds in the course of the healthcare intervention. Other decisions are more major, and can be classed as macro-decisions, such as setting up an outreach service, or withdrawing an existing provision, or changing over to a newer way of organising care. Macro-decisions tend to involve and affect more people, and take longer to complete.

Yet another consideration in decision-making is ethical decision-making, in which the five basic ethical principles, namely the value of life, goodness and rightness, justice and fairness, truth telling and honesty, and individual freedom need to be heeded. These concepts are examined in most books (e.g. Singleton and McLaren, 1995; Thiroux and Krasemann, 2007) on healthcare ethics, and they explain in detail how these principles apply. Briefly they mean:

The value of life	Refers to enhancing patients' health and well-being.
Goodness and rightness	Refers to actions that are socially seen as doing good, and what is right, for those in their care.
Justice and fairness	Being fair and just towards all patients and ensuring that they are justly protected from incompetent practice.
Truth telling and honesty	Ensuring correct practices are transparently transmitted.
Individual freedom	Promoting choice.

Creativity in decision-making

Each instance of decision-making and problem-solving could present opportunities for growth and development, as although problems may be encountered with relative annoyance at first as they disrupt plans, they may also present scope for developing new knowledge and skills, or even changing attitudes. Under the significance of decisions made by healthcare practitioners, it is clear that several decisions have interpersonal implications.

Where decision-making and problem-solving involve dealing with novel situations, novel actions may be required, which would involve thinking creatively. There are different and sequential ways of being creative. Marriner-Tomey (2004) suggests that being creative entails five stages, which are:

1 the felt need to be creative in relation to a decision or problem situation;
2 preparation – which involves exploring several possible solutions;
3 incubation – is a period for pondering over solutions after all potential solutions have been identified;
4 illumination – when the most logical or preferred solution emerges; and
5 verification – when the solution is implemented, tested, monitored, refined and evaluated.

The preparation stage can entail group or team work where appropriate, and utilise group techniques such as information sharing, focused case analysis, ideas generation exercises and SWOT analyses. Whether situations are dealt with individually or in groups, we also need to be aware of various factors that can either encourage or block creativity in practice settings.

Creative people tend to view problems as new challenges that provide scope for learning, they are always open to alternative views and lines of action, are much more flexible and adaptable, and are enthusiastic about novel ventures and openings. They do not see authority as the final, definite and only perspective, and are keen to be part of new developments. How the roles of individual team members combine for effective decision-making in care delivery is discussed in Chapter 10 under team roles in the context of inter-professional and inter-agency working.

Systematic approaches to decision-making and problem-solving

Following on from the notion that novel decision-making and problem-solving situations in particular can also present scope for being creative, it therefore follows that some decisions the DCM makes might involve innovative actions. Consequently decisions can be seen as innovative decisions, otherwise they might be routine decisions or adaptive decisions.

Types of decisions

Routine decisions involve using established rules, policies or procedures, such as what to do if a member of staff makes a drug error, a complaint is received, or a mental health patient who is detained under the Mental Health Act leaves the organisation, as for these, there is a policy or guidelines to follow. Routine decisions are often made by more junior managers as the actions to take are well-established.

Adaptive decisions are made when both problems and alternative solutions are some-what unusual or only partly understood, such as a patient admitted with an unknown identity, or with a health problem that does not normally occur at a certain age. Ways of dealing with similar previous situations may be adapted.

Innovative decisions are made when problems are unusual, unclear or unprecedented, and creative novel solutions are required, such as how to cater for the healthcare needs of the increasing number of over-85s in a particular locality, or for a new group of immigrant workers living in the area.

Managerial decisions include both individual and organisational processes, as the decisions made affect both staff and systems within the organisation. For example, if it is decided that a dietician should set up a weight self-management programme for obese patients of a general practitioner surgery, then both organisational and individual actions have to be considered. At organisational level, there will be a need to establish the availability of necessary resources such as salary for the dietician, rooms where they can meet the patients on a regular basis, probably administrative support, a referral system for the practice nurse and the general practitioner to refer patients to the dietician, and details of anticipated patient outcomes. At individual level, they need to ensure they have full knowledge of the physiological and psychological interface of obesity, and the skills to run the programme.

 Action point 4.2 – Routine, adaptive and innovative decisions

Refer back to the list of decisions that you made in response to Action point 4.1, and consider which of the decisions were routine decisions, which were adaptive decisions, and which were innovative. Mark them as R, A or I accordingly.
   Consider the processes that you have utilised to reach the final decisions.

Systematic approaches to decision-making entail ascertaining the types of situations being encountered and the decision-making techniques utilised, along with group decision-making, as well as exploring the implications of non-decisions.

Probability analysis

With flattening management structures, increasingly, more decisions and accountability are devolved to individual healthcare practitioners. However, although several decisions are made with the expectation of a high degree of certainty of achieving the anticipated outcomes, there is almost always some risk of the outcome not being achieved. Thus routine decisions made by healthcare practitioners and DCMs should present a 'high certainty' of being the correct decision, and low risk of being incorrect. Decisions are made under conditions of certainty when alternatives and conditions surrounding alternatives are known, and when therefore decisions can be made with a fairly good knowledge of the likely consequences.

DCMs make decisions in expectation of particular outcomes. The likelihood of achievement of the particular outcomes might be high, medium or low. If a patient is suspected of having an infection, then the decision may be to administer an appropriate course of antibiotics in the expectation that it will clear the infection. However, despite research evidence, it is not guaranteed 100 per cent that this outcome will be achieved as various other variables might come into play. In social situations, the likelihood of the achievement of outcomes may again be high but would be even less certain. This is referred to as decision based on probability by Hellriegel et al. (2002), and involves probability analysis before making the decision. For every decision made, the DCM needs to weigh up or endeavour to gauge the probability of the decision achieving the anticipated goal, and the risks being taken.

Adaptive decisions involve moderate degrees of certainty and risk. Innovative decisions can involve high uncertainty and high risk. A number of healthcare management decisions, such as staffing the unit for the next 24 hours, are based on probability estimates (expressed as a percentage), generally made under conditions of some risk that the actions might not succeed.

In the above examples, the decisions based on research, and facts and figures can be referred to as having objective probability, and therefore more likely to be the right decisions, and those based on less empirical evidence as having subjective probability, as they are often based on personal judgement.

Hellriegel et al. (2002) note that in situations where decisions involve more objective probabilities, as in routine decisions, there is more certainty of that being the right decision, but where they are made with subjective probabilities as in innovative or adaptive decisions, there would be less certainty. Decisions are made under conditions of uncertainty when all alternative options, the attendant risks and likely consequences of each option are not known (also known as 'limited control decisions' – Shoup, 2000). Figure 4.1 illustrates this.

Other types of decision-making include 'delayed action decisions' (Shoup, 2000:115) such as awarding a pay rise but delaying payment by six months. They can be 'provisional decisions', which implies decisions contingent upon certain pre-requisite, such as booking annual leave 12 months in advance – the pre-requisite being that staffing and the amount of work remain stable.

Approaches to decision-making

There are a number of alternative approaches to the decision-making process. For instance, rational decision-making which is a decision-making model based on logical, well-grounded rational choices that maximise the achievement of objectives. It constitutes what can be considered to be logical decisions. For example, if the road is very busy, then the pedestrian may decide to cross the road at the designated

Figure 4.1 *Types of decisions based on risk and certainty*

Routine decisions	Adaptive decisions	Innovative decisions
More objectivity		More subjectivity
Certainty ←——————— Certainty continuum		———————→ Uncertainty
Low risk ←——————— Risk continuum		———————→ High risk

crossing point; if an in-patient who is undergoing a structured rehabilitation programme requests permission to spend the weekend at home, then the decision to
grant this will be based on a number of factors which may include consulting
appropriate personnel.

Another perspective is the optimum approach, which constitutes selecting an
approach that aims to produce the best possible outcome for all parties involved.
Otherwise, a pessimistic approach to decision-making can be taken whereby the
worst possible outcomes for each alternative are compared and the least objectionable
one is chosen. For instance, if the choices of decisions between admitting an older
person with a fractured tibia from the Accident and Emergency department to a
hospital 25 miles away, or waiting in an admission unit on a trolley for a bed to become
available at the same hospital, or admitting to a mixed sex unit with a reasonable level
of privacy at the same hospital, the third alternative might be the least objectionable.
This is decision-making through screening out the unacceptable options and choosing
the best one from the remaining options.

Another approach is the political decision-making model which is a process in
which the particular interests and objectives of powerful stakeholders or allies
influence the decisions made by individuals.

Decision-making based on knowledge and intuition

 Action point 4.3 – Basis for decisions made

Refer back to Action point 4.1, and consider item 'b' with regard to whether the
decisions were made consciously or subconsciously. Then think of the basis on which
each of the decisions were made. More specifically, were the decisions based on
thorough knowledge of facts, or on intuition?

Hamm (1988) suggests that we make decisions about a situation based somewhere
on a continuum that has knowledge from empirical studies at one end, and intuition
at the other. It depends also on the time available, and therefore if for instance, when
less time is available as in a critical situation, then intuitive approaches are also relied
upon – see Figure 4.2.

In healthcare, decisions are based predominantly on knowledge from
cognitive modes 1 to 4 on Hamm's cognitive continuum, that is, on research evidence,
quasi-experiments (e.g. clinical audits), and system-aided judgement (e.g. by receiving
and using pathology laboratory results available electronically and accessed directly
from the practice setting's computer). These components generally apply to what
Hamm refers to as well-structured situations. The 'analysis' mode is a slower process,
comprising of careful scrutiny of available knowledge, conscious and consistent, usually quite accurate, and using organisational principles. Analysis involves breaking
things down for greater understanding, whereas intuition retains wholeness.

For less structured situations, peer-aided judgement and intuition tend to be used.
It is suggested that experienced professionals use 'intuitive judgement' more often,

Figure 4.2 *Hamm's (1988) cognitive continuum*

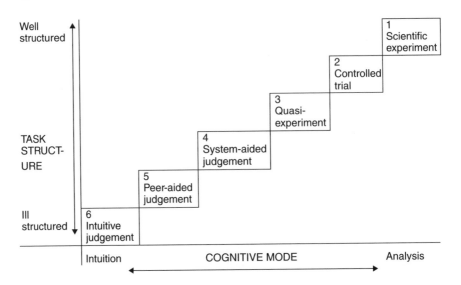

and with more self-confidence. The intuitive mode involves rapid unconscious information processing (Thompson, 1999) that combines and averages the available information, is low in consistency and is moderately accurate.

Hamm (1988) indicates that a rational intuitive approach to decision-making is primarily determined by: (i) the complexity of task structure, (ii) the ambiguity of the task and (iii) the nature of presentation of the task. If the task is complex, unfamiliar and the time available is limited, then intuitive approaches are used (Thompson, 1999). When ample clues about the situation are available, which is therefore less ambiguous, and the situation can be addressed as sub-tasks, then analytical approaches can be taken.

Problems can be solved using (i) knowledge (including information), (ii) experience and (iii) intuition. Clearly, DCMs have to base as many of their clinical decisions on research knowledge as possible. Looking back at Action point 4.1, consider the nature or types of knowledge base on which you made your decisions. Professional knowledge can also be viewed from Carper's (1978) patterns of knowing perspective, each of these 'patterns' being seen as equally important for clinical practice and for developing further knowledge. These patterns of knowing are:

(a) **Empirical knowledge**   Knowledge from traditional science viewing reality as something that can be measured, tested and authenticated

(b) **Ethical knowledge**   Knowledge based on morals and philosophy, and that which cannot usually be tested

(c) **Aesthetic knowledge**   Knowledge based on sensitivity and intuition

(d) **Personal knowledge**   Knowing of oneself in influencing one's practice.

In a study exploring whether nurses use research to inform decision-making, Thompson (2002) found that although colleagues are the more immediate source of information on which to base decisions, they are also a source of research knowledge and useful networks. However, decisions made by DCMs are also influenced by experience and intuition, which are in fact based on the healthcare practitioner's own accumulated repertoire of knowledge and mastery over its manipulation, production and application (Schon, 1995; Dearlove 1997).

Intuitive knowledge is related to patterns of personal knowledge, and tends to refer to sudden perceptions or realisation of a pattern, or 'cause and effect' in an apparently disjointed set of situations. Furthermore, Benner (2001) suggests that novices tend to prefer to use rules and guidelines, that is, practical knowledge, while 'expert' healthcare practitioners tend to use intuition more.

Group (or consensus) decision-making

Another systematic approach to decision-making is group decision-making. When a decision is made to choose from and implement, say a health clinic for asylum seekers or an evening clinic for all patients, then such a decision is better taken as a group after the appropriate discussions, as co-operation by all staff may be required.

Of course decisions that are made at strategic level are made by structured committees. However, although group decision-making is generally preferred because of its democratic element, consensus and increased commitment, it might also have its limitations or drawbacks, in that they are more time consuming, and can lower the decisiveness that leaders are expected to manifest. Furthermore, Alexander (1997) notes that professional decision-making is becoming increasingly complex and anxiety-causing for healthcare workers, as the needs of individual patients have to be balanced against resource constraints, the increase in litigation and consumer awareness and expectation.

Furthermore, referring to the contingency model of leadership, decision-making approaches are also dependent upon leadership styles as to whether they are autocratic, consultative or laissez-faire for instance.

Another aspect of decision-making is related to the quality of decisions. On evaluating the decision chosen for a particular situation, the DCM might decide that it was not the best decision, which could have been due to shortage of time and resources, for instance. Marquis and Huston (2006) also suggest that the quality of decisions could be less than desirable due to lack of clear objectives, faulty data gathering, lack of self-awareness, generating limited alternatives, faulty logic and/or inability to choose the appropriate decision and act.

Problem-solving methods

As problem-solving is a slightly different concept from decision-making, there are distinct methods of solving problems to choose from. Those related to staff conflict will be discussed shortly. Consider in the meantime the following situations.

- While performing a medical intervention, a new doctor is being rude to a member of your team.
- You arrive on duty and find that one of your colleagues who should be on duty has just rung in sick.

What are the processes that the DCM would go through to resolve the issues, and what are the factors that determine the final decision? In management problem-solving comprises taking a systematic set of actions that involve careful consideration of all variables to resolve, or to avert a problematic situation.

Thus, on encountering a problem, the DCM may have a range of choices of actions to choose from to solve it. For instance, if the problem is outside their competence or responsibility, the DCM may pass the problem on to relevant other personnel. Alternatively, they may need to seek expert advice (i.e. further knowledge) before taking further action. They may decide to share the issue with the team to explore the problem and suggest the most suitable solutions. Past experiences and intuition can be used to resolve problems, whereupon previously successfully used problem-solving methods might be used.

Yet another alternative is that the DCM may decide to ignore the problem depending on its significance in the hope that it solves itself. Problems can be solved on their own when the problem runs its natural course. For instance, a mentor may decide not to formally assess a student who is struggling to meet his/her practice outcomes as the student may be already aware of this, and taking actions to achieve the outcomes. However, problems being solved on their own are rare, as usually some action has to be taken by someone to resolve it. Therefore this is a dangerous problem-solving strategy, and in the example provided, delayed action could result in other repercussions.

At times, the trial-and-error method may be used by DCMs with lesser management experience, whereupon they try different solutions until one works. However, the traditional problem-solving method, as identified by several authors – including Bond and Holland (1998) and Marquis and Huston (2006), and which can also be represented as a uni-directional path or as a problem-solving spiral comprises:

- Define the problem
- Gather information
- Analyse the information
- Develop solutions
- Select a solution
- Implement the solution
- Evaluate the solution.

Nonetheless, further consideration of problem-solving reveals that it requires identifying and defining the problem in the first place, and thereafter utilising decision-making strategies. In problem-solving, the DCM can also take into account the Plan-Do-Study-Act (PDSA) cycle (Institute of Healthcare Improvement, 2007) which is an action-orientated learning method that comprises implementing new actions by planning, trying it out, observing the results and acting on what has been learnt. This method is also discussed in the context of quality assurance in Chapter 5, and the management of change in Chapter 6.

However, 'experimentation' is another alternative problem-solving method suggested by Sullivan and Decker (2005), which entails taking a more rigorous approach that involves empirical testing of a theory, hypothesis or hunch to determine the most appropriate solutions, including pilot projects.

Competing challenges and conflict in practice settings

The decision-making and problem-solving managerial roles of the DCM include pre-empting problems, and taking action to avert or resolve them when they do occur. The DCM needs to recognise these challenges, that there are times when things do not go smoothly, and that there can be disagreements between individuals or groups. Such disagreements can manifest themselves as open disturbances, or as latent conflict situations.

Conflict in practice settings – what are the causes?

Conflict is part of normal organisational life. There are several reasons for conflict, not least because of the numerous decisions that are continually being made by different healthcare practitioners in the day-to-day provision of healthcare in various departments. Another perspective is that each employee and sub-group in the organisation is in some way different from one other, and each have their own beliefs, perceptions, thoughts, expectations and aspirations about the employing organisation, and therefore there are likely to be situations when views differ markedly, and now and again clash with one another. These can lead to disagreements that require attention to restore equilibrium. For instance, some employees may be given 'term time contracts' under *Improving Working Lives Standard* (DH, 2000b), and therefore are away from work during summer, for instance, but this may be resented by those who do not have young families and yet would also like to take extended time away from work during summer.

The word *'conflict'* originates from the Latin word 'confligere', which means clash, contend, fight or struggle (Brown, 2002:484). It could mean 'don't agree', argument, different priorities, different attitudes, different perceptions, ineffective or lack of communication, for instance.

Conflict is generally defined as the internal or external discord that results from differences in ideas, values or feelings between two or more people (e.g. Marquis and Huston, 2006), or as deliberate behaviour intended to obstruct the achievement of some other person's goals (Mullins, 2007). Conflict can be based on the incompatibility of goals and arises from opposing behaviours. It can occur at individual, group or organisational level, and there can be negative or positive outcomes from any particular conflict.

Incidence and sources of conflict

Examples of conflict that could occur in practice settings include:

- two members of staff wanting to be nominated for the same next professional development course;
- staff being told by their managers that they must do internal rotation between day and night shifts, but this clashes with several individuals' domestic lives;
- banning overtime pay;
- being asked to lead a form of therapy for which you have not had training;
- an older patient is kept in hospital for social rather than ill-health reasons; and
- a manager wants a patient discharged home quickly, so that the bed can be free for use by a patient waiting in the Accident and Emergency Department, but the healthcare practitioner feels that more time is needed for certain facilities to be in place to ensure a safe discharge.

Various potential sources of organisational conflict can be identified. They can be caused by differences in perception; limited resources; departmentalisation and specialisation; or inequitable treatment, for instance Mullins (2007). Bryans and Cronin (1983) identify the potential sources of organisational conflict as:

1　differences between corporate and individual goals;
2　conflict between different departments or groups within the organisation;
3　conflict between the formal and the informal organisation (discussed in Chapter 2);
4　conflict between manager and managed;
5　conflict between individual and job; and
6　conflict between individuals.

 Action point 4.4 – Potential sources of organisational conflict

Think of real-life examples of sources of conflict in your own healthcare organisation for each potential source of organisational conflict identified by Bryans and Cronin, and make some notes on this in the grid format below.

Instances of potential sources of organisational conflict	
Differences between corporate and individual goals	
Between different departments or groups	
Between the formal and the informal organisation	
Between manager and managed	
Between individual and job	
Between individuals	

You should have been able to think of a few examples of sources of conflict in your healthcare organisation. There are also different types of conflict that the DCM could encounter during their normal day-to-day management activities. Conflict can therefore exist between groups (intergroup conflict), between individuals (interpersonal conflict), within the individual (intrapersonal conflict), or within a group (intragroup conflict). Conflict can also be competitive conflict, or disruptive conflict.

However, conflict does not have to be a bad thing, as although it can have negative effects, it can also produce growth, depending on how it is managed. On the other hand, too little disagreement could result in organisational stasis; but too much conflict can reduce the organisation's effectiveness.

The conflict process

How does conflict progress from the time it is initially felt by one or the other party? Filley (1975) identifies five stages of the conflict process, which can be represented diagrammatically as follows:

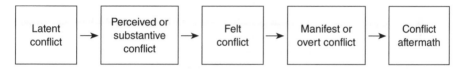

In the *latent conflict stage*, certain antecedents such as staff shortage or budget cuts persist, and conditions are 'ripe' for conflict. During the *perceived or substantive conflict stage* issues start to be explored, and if there is substantial disagreement between the two parties, then *felt conflict* is experienced. At this stage, the conflict is emotionalised, and hostility, fear and mistrust prevail. In the *manifest or overt conflict stage* action has to be taken to resolve the conflict; and in the *conflict aftermath stage*, positive or negative outcomes ensue for the two parties.

When there is conflict in a practice setting, this is detectable by the personnel in the setting, as symptoms of (potential or actual) conflict such as: irritability, mistrust, raised voices or shouting, low morale, suspiciousness, lack of communication, some staff being absent or 'off-sick' frequently and staff being unapproachable.

Responding to, and resolving conflict

 Action point 4.5 – Response to conflict: case study and alternative approaches

Case study

You are an experienced band 5 healthcare practitioner, and you are encouraged to apply for the band 6 vacancy that has been advertised. You have the required experience in the specialism and know you can do the job. You apply, get interviewed, but the job is given to someone else who is external to the organisation,

Action point 4.5 – Continued

has less years' experience but has a university degree, which you do not have. You feel you have been 'led up the garden path', and furthermore, will have to help the new person settle in.

From the case study, first identify your initial reactions, and secondly see if you can think of alternative approaches to the situation. Thirdly, consider what are the possible positive outcomes, and the possible negative outcomes of the particular conflict?

Your initial reaction to the situation might be resentment towards your employer, or a philosophical reaction such as 'some you win, some you lose'. Nonetheless, the likely negative outcomes of conflict might include feeling defeated and demeaned, with consequent lowered self-esteem, creating a cold social atmosphere of mistrust and suspicion, loss of motivation, sickness, and even leaving the employment, resulting in an increase in employee turnover. There can be a loss of self-confidence, for instance whether to apply for similar position. Employees might find it difficult to take orders or instructions from the other person, there could be resistance to team work, and individuals and groups might become more self-interested.

There are various likely positive outcomes from the above case study. To start with, the vacancy is filled, and therefore the unit is back to a full complement of staff. Both parties could learn new skills or knowledge from each other and gain new perspectives. It is also an opportunity to identify CPD needs based on why you did not get the job, and enable you to seek support for further professional development. Both have the opportunity to network and make a new professional acquaintance. You can apply for a different job, and see this as an interview experience. You could go for post-interview counselling, to receive constructive critique of your performance at the interview and suggestions on how you can learn from the experience.

General positive outcomes of conflict that could ensue include:

- increased problem-solving ability through being forced to search for new approaches;
- other underlying problems being brought to the surface and getting resolved;
- individuals' views getting clarified, and protocols being established;
- stimulation of interest and re-motivation; and
- an opportunity to test own abilities further.

However, conflict tends to cause stress, hardening of attitudes, and a tendency to be rigid and as individuals, and we tend to develop habitual ways of reacting to conflict situations.

Resolving conflict – goals and strategies

Pedler et al. (2001) note that there are five particular modes or styles of conflict resolution: competing, collaborating, compromising, avoiding and accommodating – see Figure 4.3. Where there is conflict between two parties the mode of resolution depends upon the two basic dimensions of conflict situations, which are:

1   how assertive or unassertive each party is in pursuing their own goals;
2   how co-operative or uncooperative each party is.

Figure 4.3 *Modes or styles of conflict resolution (Pedler et al. 2007)*

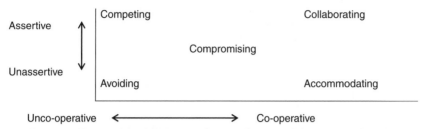

Pedler, Burgoyne, Boydell, from A Manager's Guide to Self Development (5th edn, 2007)
@ McGraw-Hill Education. Reproduced by permission

If both parties are highly assertive and uncooperative, this reflects a competing (battling) style. But if both parties are highly unassertive and uncooperative, then they could avoid facing the conflict, as if it does not exist. If both parties are highly assertive and highly co-operative, then they will be using the collaborating mode. At times, the two parties may adopt different styles or modes of resolution in a particular conflict. Resolving conflict is an interactive situation in which styles are mutually reciprocal. The style you adopt will affect the style your opponent adopts, and vice versa. Disjunction and difficulty in resolving conflict occurs if one party is, say, in competing mode while the other is in avoiding mode.

 Action point 4.6 – My reaction to conflict

Use the above illustration by Pedler et al. (2001) to identify how you have personally reacted to a particular conflict situation in which you have been involved. Did you react assertively or unassertively, co-operatively or uncooperatively? How did the other party react? Was your actual response the same as your initial reaction?

The style of resolving conflict varies with such factors as the nature of the current interaction between you and the other party. It may be affected by contingent issues such as power, urgency and clarity of goals. However, by identifying any habitual responses you may have in certain situations and observing the responses these produce in others, you can obtain a clearer picture of yourself. After identifying your own style(s) or modes and the responses generated in others, you still have scope to select the response you feel is the most appropriate one.

Managing conflict

On encountering conflict situations, DCMs can draw on various available strategies, such as the modes or styles of conflict resolution suggested by Pedler et al. (2001) noted above. Sullivan and Decker (2005) suggest that other strategies for conflict management are:

Negotiation – The conflicting parties discuss the issues and give and take on particular elements.

Confrontation	– The problem is openly discussed by all parties involved.
Win-win strategy	– Strategy that focuses on goals or the welfare of both parties, and attempts are made to meet the needs of both parties; is also known as joint-welfare choice
Win-lose strategy	– One party is determined to win, and the other has to submit or lose.
Lose-lose strategy	– Strategy in which neither side wins, nor settlement reached, and is unsatisfactory for both sides.
Partisan choice	– Attending to the needs of only one party.

For conflict to be resolved successfully, it is essential that each party is clear about their goals and objectives. If the goals of the two parties are diametrically opposed to one another, then a mutually beneficial (i.e. joint-welfare or win-win) outcome might be more difficult to achieve.

Clinical managers realise that conflict is a natural and inevitable process in organisations, and often, it also comprises a precursor for change. Conflict can be seen as the cutting edge of change (Yoder-Wise, 2003). Resolving conflict is an interactive and dynamic process, and can be positive or negative. Responses to conflict situations include resolving them by analysing a variety of alternatives as positive opportunities, by identifying goals and particular strategies, and not seeing them as negative obligations.

Overall, dealing with conflict, is also related to coping strategies, which can be facilitated through clinical supervision for instance, which is discussed in Chapter 8. Healthcare practitioners must not allow themselves to feel stressed by conflict situations, but to treat them as challenges that comprise opportunities for learning from events.

Guidelines for effective decision-making, problem-solving and conflict management

The following constitute guidelines for effective decision-making, problem-solving and conflict management in practice settings.

- Accept decision-making, problem-solving and conflict management as normal management activities, and see them as opportunities for positive outcomes and learning.
- Do not delay decision-making, problem-solving and conflict management unduly, as delays can lead to unnecessary complications.
- Use systematic approaches to decision-making, problem-solving and conflict management whenever possible.
- Be clear about the goals of each situation prior to taking interventional actions.
- Allow plenty of space and scope for individual and teams to develop creativity when faced with issues.

Chapter summary

This chapter has explored the decision-making and problem-solving function of DCMs. Key components of these concepts were examined, which include:

- day-to-day personal and professional decisions and their significance, including instances of decisions that healthcare practitioners make during the course of a day; and why decision-making and problem-solving are important clinical management functions;
- what decision-making and problem-solving are, together with distinctions between them, micro- and macro-decisions , and creativity in decision-making;
- systematic approaches to decision-making and problem-solving, including types of decisions, probability analysis, approaches to decision-making, decisions based on knowledge or intuition, group decision-making, and problem-solving methods;
- competing challenges and conflicts in practice settings, including what they are, incidents and sources of conflict, and the conflict process;
- responding to conflict, and resolving conflicts through goal setting, and using strategies of conflict management; and
- guidelines for effective decision-making, that is, applying the principles of effective decision-making and problem-solving.

FIVE Ensuring quality in healthcare

Introduction

The provision of high quality healthcare is becoming increasingly challenging with rising consumer expectations, increasing technological advances, demographic changes and budgetary constraints. Healthcare providers need to be competitive to attract patients and ensure the financial viability of their respective organisations. The DCM has a vital role in maximising the use of resources and ensuring the best outcomes for patients in their practice setting. Quality in healthcare encompasses ensuring safety and that the patient comes to no harm, while also ensuring that a high standard of care is achieved. This chapter focuses on quality, patient safety and the patient experience. The concept of total quality management (TQM) will be explored together with a number of models and tools of quality assurance.

Chapter objectives

On completion of this chapter, you will be able to:

- define and distinguish between quality, quality assurance and related concepts;
- identify the various component parts that sit under the Clinical Governance umbrella and evaluate their significance for the role of the DCM;
- explore the principles of customer care and apply them within your practice setting to ensure a good patient experience; and
- discuss various strategies for quality improvement and quality monitoring and apply them within your practice setting.

Since the inception of *The NHS Plan* (DH, 2000a), the NHS has experienced investment and growth in both its staffing and facilities. Coupled with recent reform, the NHS over the last decade has realised reduced waiting times and ongoing improvements in efficiency. *High Quality Care for All* (Darzi report) (DH, 2008) sets out a vision of an NHS that has 'quality of care at its heart'. The definition of quality adopted encompasses three key areas: 'clinically effective, personal and safe'. This policy document sets out the requirement for the publication of 'quality accounts' which will include a number of metrics from mortality rates to patient satisfaction. The chapter will now explore the concept of quality and strategies for quality assurance.

Defining quality

It is often stated that quality as a concept is difficult to define as all individuals have their own interpretation of its meaning. Quality care provision is care delivery that meets a certain standard of excellence that is acceptable to both staff and patients. There are a plethora of definitions in existence, but they are dependent upon two sets of factors: intrinsic and extrinsic; the former relates to values, beliefs, attitudes and self-knowledge, and the latter to time, money, people and other resources and so forth.

 Action point 5.1 – What quality care means to me

Consider what 'quality care' means to you. If a close family member became a patient within your practice setting, what type of service would you like them to receive? Focus your thoughts around the four areas identified within the Darzi review (DH, 2007a), namely:

1 Fair
2 Personalised
3 Effective
4 Safe.

In achieving quality care it is necessary to both agree on the definition of quality, and how to measure quality. The chapter will now address quality assurance, and the monitoring and evaluation of quality.

Quality assurance refers to assuring the receiver of an identified degree of excellence of service, goods, or standard of care that is continually monitored through actively sought relevant data. The level of achievement of quality is measured and actions are taken to correct identified deficiencies.

TQM

TQM is a strategy to get an organisation working to its maximum effectiveness and efficiency (NHSME, 1993). It does this by challenging traditional ways of working and encouraging organisations to adopt innovative practices. In a mature TQM organisation:

- everything is driven by its customers' needs;
- a highly trained and motivated workforce continually seeks better ways of working;
- change is based on measured fact and monitored in a continuous cycle of improvement;
- errors are relentlessly traced and eliminated; and
- hands-on management drives the quest for quality.

 Action point 5.2 – Measuring quality of care

- Consider reasons why the quality of care provided within your practice setting needs to be measured.
- What methods are utilised to measure the quality of care delivered in your practice setting?

Quality assurance frameworks

There are several published frameworks or models of quality assurance that can be used for measuring and monitoring quality assurance. These include:

- Clinical Governance
- Maxwell's elements of quality
- Donabedian's structure, process and outcome model.

Clinical Governance

Clinical Governance is a framework through which NHS organisations are accountable for continuously improving the quality of their services and safeguarding high standards of care by creating an environment in which excellence in clinical care will flourish (DH, 1998). Clinical Governance was developed to ensure accountability for the safe delivery of healthcare.

Clinical Governance can be viewed as an umbrella term for a number of key components that collectively combine to facilitate the delivery of safe high quality care. The component parts are all equally relevant while also having an interdependent relationship. Aspects contained within the framework of Clinical Governance are discussed within the various chapters of the book. As identified by the Clinical Governance Support Team (2007), the component parts of Clinical Governance include:

- Patient, public and carer involvement – analysis of patient-professional involvement and interaction, and strategy, planning and delivery of care, as discussed in Chapter 9.
- Strategic capacity and capability – planning, communication and governance arrangements, and cultural behaviour aspects, as discussed in Chapter 1.
- Risk Management – incident reporting, infection control, prevention and control of risk (discussed later in the chapter).
- Staff management and performance – recruitment, workforce planning, appraisals, as discussed in Chapter 7.
- Education, training and continuous professional development – professional re-validation, management development, confidentiality and data protection, as discussed in Chapter 11.
- Clinical effectiveness – clinical audit management, planning and monitoring, learning through research and audit (discussed later in the chapter).
- Information management – patient records and other data (discussed later in the chapter).
- Communication – patient and public, external partners, internal, board and organisation-wide, as discussed in Chapters 1, 9 and 10.
- Leadership – throughout the organisation, including board, chair and non-executive directors, chief executive and executive directors, managers and clinicians, as discussed in Chapter 2.
- Team working – within the service, senior managers, clinical and multi-disciplinary teams, and across organisations, as discussed in Chapter 10.

All these components are examined either in this chapter or in other chapters in this book. The key component parts explored next include clinical effectiveness, audit, risk management, information management and benchmarking.

Clinical effectiveness

Clinical effectiveness is concerned with clinical interventions that are based on the best available evidence and applying such interventions to real life conditions. Clinical effectiveness is doing the **right** thing in the **right** way for the **right** patients at the **right** time (RCN, 1996). This involves getting **evidence** of what works in everyday clinical practice and evaluating its effect on patient care. Clinical guidelines are one vehicle by which clinical effectiveness can be addressed through the provision of evidence-based recommendations for good practice (Duff, 1998). As mentioned earlier in the chapter, clinical effectiveness comprises a component part of Clinical Governance that provides a mechanism to evaluate whether clinical effectiveness is being achieved.

Clinical audit

A clinical audit comprises a systematic assessment or estimation of the process or outcome of a clinical activity, to determine whether it is:

- *Effective:* making progress towards particular goals
- *Efficient:* achieving a particular target with the least effort
- *Economic:* achieving a successful outcome with the minimum cost

Essentially audit measures what healthcare practitioners are doing against what they should be doing. Clinical audit involves systematically looking at the procedures used for diagnosis, care and treatment, examining how associated resources are used and investigating the effect care has on the outcome and quality of life for the patient (DH, 1993). Conversely, research is concerned with the identification of best practice, whereas audit establishes whether agreed best practice is being followed, and according to Smith (1992) 'Research is concerned with discovering the right thing to do; audit with ensuring that it is done right.'

There are two types of audit:

1 Retrospective – examines what happened after the episode of care has been completed.
2 Concurrent – examines what is happening at the time it is taking place.

An example of a retrospective audit could include the examination of case notes to establish compliance with standards of record keeping. An example of a concurrent audit can include hand washing where the auditor monitors the use of hand gel as people enter and exit the practice setting.

A range of methods used to collect evidence about the quality of care in concurrent and retrospective audit is provided in Table 5.1.

Risk management

Risk is part of everyday life and is similarly part and parcel of clinical practice. Throughout our daily lives we make a number of decisions that have an element of risk associated with them such as crossing the road and driving our cars. Clinical risk

Table 5.1 *Audit data collection methods*

Method	Concurrent	Retrospective
Observation	✓	—
Checklist	✓	✓
Documentation audit	✓	✓
Questionnaire	✓	✓
Interview	✓	✓
Case review	✓	✓

management is a proactive approach that involves:

- risk identification;
- risk assessment;
- taking action to reduce the likelihood of the risk occurring; and
- monitoring the outcomes and reassessing the level of risk as appropriate.

A number of variables have been identified that can increase our risk of developing a deep vein thrombosis or sustaining a fall. The risk of a patient having a fall, for example, can be reduced by completing a validated risk assessment to establish the level of risk, together with an intervention plan commensurate with the level of risk identified. Interventions can include addressing both intrinsic and extrinsic factors. Intrinsic factors in this example can include co morbidities, the presence of a cognitive impairment and polypharmacy, and extrinsic factors can include environmental factors such as wet floors and poor lighting.

Within the Clinical Governance Framework, incident reporting is utilised as a mechanism to monitor adverse events and near misses, to identify trends and to ensure that the organisation learns from the incidents that occur and is responsive to implement actions for risk reduction. The DCM has a responsibility to ensure that team members complete risk assessments as required and that any adverse incidents or near misses are reported in accordance with the policy of the employing organisation.

Sometimes clinical staff can consider incident reporting as bureaucratic and creating more paperwork. It is important that staff do not become complacent and that incidents are always reported as this provides the opportunity for lessons to be learnt and actions taken to prevent reoccurrence. When completing an incident form it is important to record the impact on patient outcomes and care delivery.

Information management

A good standard of record keeping is imperative to support Clinical Governance and forms an essential element of the role of the DCM regardless of professional background. In order to support Clinical Governance, Sanderson (2000) identifies three key areas of information that are required:

1 Policies, protocols and guidelines to inform practice
2 Information regarding care delivery
3 Information about systems, for example, incident reporting.

Benchmarking and The Essence of Care

Benchmarking is defined as 'The practice of being humble enough to admit that someone else is better at something and being wise enough to try to learn how to match and even surpass them at it' (Ellis, 1995:25). Benchmarking encourages searching for examples of best practice from others engaged in similar practice. Whoever achieves best practice shares their methods with others.

The *Essence of Care* (DH, 2003) utilises the benchmarking process to facilitate practitioners to utilise a structured approach to sharing and comparing practice. It includes a toolkit that focuses upon the fundamentals of care and enables practitioners to identify best practice and develop action plans to improve practice. *Essence of Care* benchmarks include:

- Patient care environment
- Promoting health
- Continence and bladder and bowel care
- Personal and oral hygiene
- Food and nutrition
- Pressure ulcers
- Privacy and dignity
- Record keeping
- Safety of clients with mental health needs in acute mental health and general hospital settings
- Principles of self care.

The benchmarks have been developed for use in both health and social care settings and their use allows for customisation by individual areas to ensure that indicators are agreed that reflect best practice within the specific area of practice. Since the initial *Essence of Care* publications, several others have been published including *Essence of Care: Benchmarks for the Care Environment* (DH, 2007e) which is the eleventh in the *Essence of Care* series, and concerns the environment within which the care of patients takes place, including patients' homes.

The stages involved in *Essence of Care* benchmarking advocated by the NHS Modernisation Agency are as follows:

1 Agree best practice
2 Assess clinical area against best practice
3 Produce and implement an action plan aimed at achieving best practice
4 Review achievement towards best practice
5 Disseminate improvements and/or review action plan.

National Service Frameworks

National Service Frameworks (NSF) provide long-term strategies for the improvement of targeted aspects of care and incorporate goals that need to be achieved within specified time frames. NSFs that have been published to date include:

- Cancer
- Children

- Coronary heart disease
- Diabetes
- Long-term conditions
- Mental health
- Older people
- Paediatric intensive care
- Renal.

Maxwell's elements of quality

Maxwell (1984) identified six elements of quality as a quality assurance framework that should be contained within a quality monitoring cycle. Maxwell's model comprises 3As and 3Es, whereupon once one quality cycle is completed a further cycle should begin straight after. The model comprises:

Acceptability	Providing a service that meets the reasonable expectations of the patients and stakeholders
Accessibility	The ease with which clinical interventions and services are accessible to the patient. Constraints to access may include distance, time and lack of knowledge
Appropriateness	Providing a service which the individual or community actually needs
Effectiveness	The extent to which the intended benefits for the individual have been achieved
Efficiency	Closely related to effectiveness and considers how resources are used
Equity	Ensuring that everyone has equal access to the service being provided

At clinical level, this framework can be utilised say in pain management. If for instance the clinical team's standard is that all patients should be pain-free within ten minutes of complaining of pain, then Maxwell's model can be used to monitor whether:

- this standard is *acceptable* to the patient and the staff;
- they have *access* to the healthcare practitioners to obtain pain relieving interventions;
- the means of pain relief is *appropriate*;
- the method of pain relief is *effective* and acceptable to both parties;
- the pain relief is administered *efficiently*; and
- all patients are afforded the *same standard* of care.

Donabedian's structure, process and outcome model

Another quality assurance framework devised by Donabedian (1988) is one that consists of three sets of criteria: structure, process and outcome.

Structure criteria

The setting in which care takes place, include the people, equipment and the environment (resources), and therefore comprises:

- the physical environment and buildings;

- ancillary services – laundry, pharmacy, paramedical services, catering, laboratory services;
- equipment;
- staff – numbers, skill mix, training, expertise;
- information – agreed policies and procedures, rules and regulations; and
- organisational system.

Process criteria

Process refers to the care given by healthcare practitioners, and therefore involves the actions of assessment, planning, implementation and evaluation (in partnership with patients and relatives where appropriate). It encompasses the knowledge held by the practitioner in:

- the assessment techniques used, and methods of delivery of care and intervention;
- the healthcare organisation's procedures and clinical guidelines;
- methods of patient, relative and/or carer education and information giving;
- methods of documenting; and
- ways in which resources are used.

Outcome criteria

The specific benefits or positive results experienced by the patient, which encompass indicators of patient outcomes, such as health status, wound healing, patient satisfaction, immunisation uptake, patients' knowledge of their condition, behaviours such as successful use of equipment by patients, as well as evaluation of the competence of staff delivering care.

Monitoring quality in healthcare

Health and social care services are externally monitored to ensure that standards are achieved and that targets are met. This monitoring function is provided in a number of ways such as by PCTs through their commissioning function, Strategic Health Authorities, the Healthcare Commission and Monitor – the independent regulator for Foundation Trusts.

The Healthcare Commission

The Healthcare Commission is the independent inspection body for healthcare for both the NHS and the independent sector.* Its role is to:

- inspect the quality and value for money of healthcare and public health;
- equip patients and the public with the best possible information about the provision of healthcare; and
- promote improvements in healthcare and public health.

* From 1 April 2009 the Healthcare Commission will merge with Commission for Social Care Inspection (CSCI) to become the Care Quality Commission. The Care Quality Commission will be a new integrated regulator for health and social care bringing together existing health and social care regulators into one regulatory body, with tough new powers to ensure safe and high quality services (see website at: http://www.dh.gov.uk/en/Publicationsandstatistics/Legislation/Actsandbills/HealthandSocialCareBill/DH_080438).

The Healthcare Commission publishes an annual health check in October each year and provides assessment and performance ratings for NHS organisations. The rating addresses quality of services and the use of resources provided on a four-part scale from excellent to weak.

Standards for Better Health

In *Standards for Better Health*, the DH (2006b) sets out the quality that NHS healthcare providers are expected to meet in relation to safety, cost effectiveness, Clinical Governance, patient focus, accessible and responsive care, care environment and amenities and public health. The standards are integral to the performance assessments undertaken by the Healthcare Commission.

 Action point 5.3 – Quality in your organisation

Log on to http://www.healthcarecommission.org.uk/homepage.cfm the home page of the Healthcare Commission website. Now access the results of the annual health check for your employing organisation/local healthcare provider, and ascertain how well the organisation has performed in relation to both quality and value for money.

Patient safety

Patient safety represents an important element in the quality equation; patients who access healthcare services want to be protected from coming to any harm. Healthcare associated infections present health care providers with a major challenge. Minimising the incidence of infections such as MRSA and Clostridium Difficile, for example, require commitment from Board level and beyond. The DCM has a responsibility to ensure that staff and visitors to the clinical area adhere to policies, procedures and protocols related to the prevention of cross-infection.

The Annual Report 2005 of the Chief Medical Officer (DH, 2006e) made parallels between aviation and healthcare in relation to safety. The report highlighted how 2004 was the safest year for air travel; with the number of worldwide fatalities mirroring those of 1945. The improvement to safety relates to the rise in the number of passengers from 9 million to 1.8 billion per annum respectively. Conclusions drawn by the Chief Medical Officer from the comparative analysis of aviation and healthcare approaches to safety identified a number of key elements to the success of aviation, namely:

- Clear goal setting
- The collection of data that are useful and used to enable everyone to understand what is being looked for and the changes that are necessary
- Comprehensive and multifaceted approaches to risk management that focus upon the important issues
- Building a safety culture that is owned by everyone in the organisation
- Oversight, monitoring and clear accountabilities for action

A pilot study into adverse events in hospitalised patients in the United Kingdom identified the proportion of in-patient episodes leading to harmful adverse events to be 10 per cent, of which it was estimated that half were preventable (Vincent, 2000).

National Patient Safety Agency

The National Patient Safety Agency (NPSA) was set up in 2001 in response to the Chief Medical Officer's report *An Organisation with a Memory* (DH, 2000d). The NPSA has responsibility for the coordination of reporting of patient safety incidents, together with learning from these incidents to improve patient safety in the NHS. In 2004 the NPSA published seven steps that NHS organisations should take in order to improve patient safety. The seven steps provide a checklist for organisations to plan and measure their performance in relation to patient safety and to ensure that appropriate action is taken when things go wrong. The seven steps are:

1 Build a safety culture
2 Lead and support your staff
3 Integrate your risk management activity
4 Promote reporting
5 Involve and communicate with patients and the public
6 Learn and share safety lessons
7 Implement solutions to prevent harm.

The following two NPSA initiatives have been designed with the intention of driving the patient safety agenda forward (NPSA, 2004).

1 National Reporting and Learning System – a national patient safety incidence data collection system, was implemented by the NPSA across NHS institutions in England and Wales in 2004.
2 Root Cause Analysis (RCA) – provides a mechanism to identify the root cause of a problem or occurrence. It is predicated on the belief that the best way to solve a problem is to eliminate the cause.

World Health Organisation

In May 2007, the World Health Organisation (WHO) (2007) published nine *Patient Safety Solutions* with the aim of reducing the incidence of healthcare related harm worldwide. The nine 'solutions' in the publication are available for use by WHO Member States and focus on the following key areas:

- look-alike, sound-alike medication names;
- patient identification;
- communication during patient handovers;
- performance of correct procedure at correct body site;
- control of concentrated electrolyte solutions;
- assuring medication accuracy at transitions in care;
- avoiding catheter and tubing disconnections;
- single use of injection devices; and
- improved hand hygiene to prevent health care-associated infection.

National Health Service Litigation Authority

The National Health Service Litigation Authority (NHSLA) (2007) was established in 1995 and is the NHS body that has responsibility for handling negligence claims made against NHS bodies in England. In 2006–07, the NHSLA received 5,426 claims of clinical negligence and 3,293 claims of non-clinical negligence against NHS bodies. The functions of the NHSLA include to:

- ensure claims are dealt with consistently and with due regard to the proper interests of the NHS and its patients;
- manage the financial consequences of such claims and to advise the DH of the likely future costs;
- advise the DH on both specific and general issues arising out of claims against the NHS;
- manage and raise the standards of risk management throughout the NHS;
- assist NHS bodies to comply with the *Human Rights Act* by providing a central source of information on relevant case-law development;
- provide mechanisms for the proper, prompt and cost-effective resolution of disputes between NHS primary care organisations and those providing, or seeking to provide, services for patients; and
- provide advice about, and assistance with, litigation concerning equal pay claims involving NHS bodies in England.

Service improvement techniques

As previously stated, a current healthcare priority is to achieve high quality and efficient services. The NHS III was set up to facilitate NHS organisations to achieve the same levels of quality and efficiency as top performing organisations. The focus of the NHS III is developing and spreading new ways of working, new technology and world-class leadership to transform healthcare for patients and the public. The NHS III has identified key areas to support the NHS to minimise variations in productivity. These areas include the development of unambiguous performance indicators to demonstrate how an organisation is performing; workable solutions focusing on clinical activities; and support for Strategic Health Authorities (SHA) with commissioning, provisioning services and clinical care. Improvement techniques supported by the NHS III include 'Lean' – an improvement approach developed by Toyota to improve flow and eliminate waste, and 'Experience Based Design' – a method to capture and understand people's perspectives in order to support redesign. Examples of service improvement techniques will now be explored.

Process mapping

Process mapping utilises a workflow diagram to represent a process or series of parallel processes. The resultant process map can provide a clear picture of the activities performed, where they are undertaken and by whom. This enables the identification of bottlenecks that can be re-engineered to improve the process. Using the example of discharge planning, the process-mapper will develop a diagram that illustrates the various steps in the process. This enables the identification of delays, for example, the prescribing or dispensing of tablets to take out (TTOs). Re-engineering of the process could be achieved in a number of ways, such as the implementation of non-medical discharge, the utilisation of a discharge lounge or the operation of a traffic light discharge system so that staff are aware of the discharge status of the patients within their care.

Metrics

Metrics provide parameters for the assessment of a process, together with the procedures to undertake the assessment in order to facilitate comparative analysis of the results. The Better Metrics Project was set up by the Healthcare Commission in 2004 with the aim of improving the way that health services are measured through:

- developing metrics that are relevant to the work of clinical staff;
- identifying metrics that have a proven track record within organisations to monitor and improve performance;
- the metrics identified are categorised under clinical conditions and areas of care such as cancer and urgent care respectively. Examples of metrics within urgent care include:
  - The proportion of patients treated in an acute stroke unit.
  - The time from first entry into an acute hospital to admission to the acute stroke unit.

Healthcare providers can identify their own metrics as part of their quality monitoring and quality assurance function. Quality metrics are also beginning to be incorporated into the commissioning process and form part of contract monitoring. Quality dashboards can be agreed that include a number of metrics to monitor the achievement of organisational quality. Metrics employed within a quality dashboard could include:

- Number of clinical incidents, for example, falls, medication errors and so on.
- Number of complaints
- Number of pressure ulcers.

Lean

In recent years the NHS has adopted service improvement techniques that were developed by the Japanese car manufacturer, Toyota. Lean is a management system that aims to maximise value through improving flow in the patient journey and eliminating all forms of waste. Waste can relate to anything that does not add value to a process. For example, 'waiting', this could be for referrals, test results, TTOs, or a ward round and so on. Another example of waste is transportation; this could include the moving of patients to other clinical areas for non-clinical reasons. A further key principle of Lean is the involvement of people in change and the rede-sign process.

Releasing Time to Care: The Productive Ward

Within healthcare, comments often made by staff include 'there's not enough time' or 'we're short of staff'. A recent survey of 1,250 nurses identified that 73% of staff nurses stated that they don't spend enough time on direct patient care (NHS III, 2007b). It identified that ward-based nurses spend less than 40 per cent of their time on direct patient care. The *Releasing Time to Care: Productive Ward Programme* utilises improvement techniques, such as those already discussed, that have been tailor-made to enable nurses to improve upon key ward processes; with a resultant freeing up of time that can be redirected into focusing on patient care delivery.

This approach to service improvement is based at grass roots level and facilitates and empowers the clinical team to have ownership and take the lead. *The Productive Ward* also requires the commitment of the Trust Board to provide support to the clinical area throughout their quality improvement journey. The programme comprises of a number of modules that include how to assess the readiness of the organisation to engage in this initiative, to preparing the ward, developing ward-based measures and the provision of information. Modules that focus on key processes for the practice setting to implement include drug administration, shift handovers and patient observations.

'Root cause analysis' and the 'incident decision tree'

Root cause analysis is undertaken retrospectively and provides a methodology for the identification of causes of patient safety incidents, thereby enabling organisations to take action to prevent future occurrences. The NPSA provides a modular e-learning training programme that can be accessed on the NPSA web site.

The 'incident decision tree' has been designed by the NPSA for use following a patient safety incident. The decision tree is available on line and takes the form of a flow chart that utilises structured questions. The decision tree can be completed within about 30 minutes and can also be accessed at the NPSA website www.npsa.nhs.uk/

The patient experience

As mentioned earlier, patients expect to come to no harm from their association with healthcare professionals and services. Patients have rising expectations of healthcare which relate to their overall experiences in addition to clinical outcomes. Customer care principles are having increasing credence and the patient experience is a key component of the quality equation.

Patient satisfaction surveys

The Healthcare Commission coordinates the completion of a number of national surveys to elicit patients' perceptions and evaluations of their recent experiences of healthcare. The 2006 survey of hospital inpatients in England identified that more than 90 per cent of patients rated their care as good, very good or excellent (Healthcare Commission, 2007). Such surveys provide NHS Trusts with the opportunity to benchmark their services against the standard of services nationally. Results are presented using traffic light colours to denote high-performing Trusts, average scores and low-performing Trusts.

Action point 5.4 – Organisational performance

How aware are you regarding how your organisation fares in relation to performance outcomes and the assessment of quality?

1   Log on to the Healthcare Commission website www.healthcarecommission.org. uk/homepage.cfm and look at the performance ratings. The results are broken down into quality of services and use of resources, so consider overall how well your organisation has performed in these two areas.
2   Now look at the results of the in-patient survey and other appropriate surveys for your organisation, consider overall how well it has performed and how it compares nationally.

   Now consider your practice setting, and the information that you routinely receive to keep you appraised of how your clinical team is performing. Look at the following list of sources of information, if you do not already have access to this information then ask your manager who should be able to make it available to you:

- Complaints data and individual letters of complaint
- Number of thank you letters and commendations
- Number of clinical incidents
- Patient length of stay statistics
- Healthcare associated infection incidence
- Mortality data.

Once you have located the information, have a look through and compare it to other practice settings within your organisation, to deduce how well your practice setting performed. From studying the results, can you identify any recurring themes or key areas where you consider your practice setting can improve? If so, think about the actions that you and your colleagues can take to make a positive difference. Is this type of information routinely discussed at team briefings and departmental meetings? If not, you may want to discuss the benefits of doing so with your manager.

Improving the patient experience

Action point 5.5 – Patients' priorities

Consider if you were a patient what would your top ten priorities be? Once you have identified your priority areas, reflect upon how your practice setting or service measures up in matching your priorities. Do you consider there to be any scope for improvement? If so, think about the management and leadership principles and models that have been discussed in Chapters 2 and 3, how you can utilise these within your role as DCM to improve and monitor the patient experience within your practice setting.

Case study – Walsall Hospitals NHS Trust 'Getting Better for Patients Campaign'

Improving the patient experience is one of five strategic imperatives for Walsall Hospitals NHS Trust. In order to identify patient experience priorities, patients and staff were invited to join together to agree customer care priorities that would be developed into standards and form the measures for ongoing customer satisfaction surveys. The outcome of this diagnostic event was the identification of the top six elements that constitute a good patient experience. The top six areas identified were:

1 Effective two-way communication
2 Privacy, dignity and respect
3 Positive, professional 'can do' attitude from staff
4 Individual care and prompt attention
5 Hand washing and infection control
6 Clean and clutter-free environment.

The six priority areas were subsequently developed into the 'Six C Model' (Figure 5.1). This model provides staff with an easy way of remembering priority areas, together with diagrammatic representation of the Trust's commitment to improve the patient experience. The model was used as the basis for a 'Getting Better for Patients' campaign, where each month, for a six-month period there was an organisation-wide focus on making improvements within each of the patient priority areas in turn.

All staff and departments were invited to participate in the campaign and a 'Patient Experience Project Group' was set up to lead the developments and to monitor the progress of the campaign. Each of the Divisions with the Trust developed their individual action plans for each of the six months of the campaign. This was coupled with a number of corporate initiatives to drive the focus of quality improvement. A patient experience questionnaire focusing on the six priority areas was developed and is routinely given to all patients on their discharge. The results of this exercise are published on the Trust's intranet site each month as league tables.

 Action point 5.6 – Patient feedback

Consider each of the patient experience priorities contained within the Six C Model; discuss each of the priorities with patients in your practice setting and invite them to give you feedback regarding their experiences, together with suggestions of improvements that could be made.

Complaints

Complaints provide a further means for healthcare services to receive feedback from their patients regarding the quality of services that they receive. Complaints arise where the standard of service received by a patient or their relatives/carer falls below the standard expected. Arguably, every patient has the right to expect a good service from both the healthcare practitioners and the services from which they receive their

Figure 5.1 *Walsall Hospitals NHS Trust (2007) – Six C model*

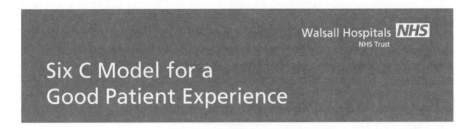

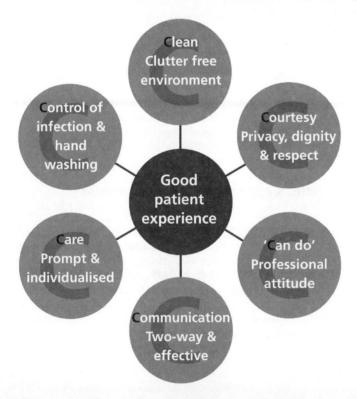

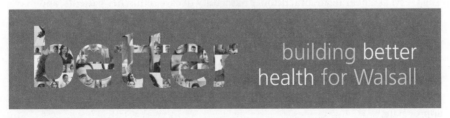

Note: Reproduced with the kind permission of Walsall Hospitals NHS Trust

care. Complainants often state that they want other people to benefit from their experiences by ensuring that the same mistakes do not happen again. Services need to learn from the experiences of complainants and take steps to ensure that root causes are addressed and remedied. In some instances the area requiring focus may be restricted to an individual service, whereas in others organisation-wide changes may need to be made to policies, processes and systems.

A framework of principles has been developed by the Parliamentary and Health Service Ombudsman (2007) with the aim of providing statements of what public bodies should achieve to ensure good administration and customer focus. The principles identified are:

- Getting it right
- Being customer focused
- Being open and accountable
- Acting fairly and proportionately
- Putting things right
- Seeking continuous improvement.

The consultation document *Making Experiences Count* (DH, 2007f) proposes a single system for the management of complaints for both health and social care. This includes focus on local resolution with greater responsibility for Trust Boards and senior managers.

 Action point 5.7 – Responding to a complaint

Ask your manager for a copy of a letter of complaint, together with a copy of the response that was forwarded to the complainant. Read the complaint and make a note of the issues raised. Think about the issues and identify any emerging themes, for example 'communication' within which to categorise the key areas raised.

Now read the letter of response to the complainant. What lessons can be learnt from the complaint? What actions can be implemented within the clinical area to ensure that the key issues are addressed? What actions could be implemented organisation-wide to address the issues identified?

Whistle blowing

The DCM as a healthcare practitioner has a duty of care to his/her patients, and needs to work within the code of conduct governed by their respective professional body. There are a number of mechanisms available to the DCM to raise any concerns that they may have about patient safety and standards and quality of care. These can include raising issues at team meetings, discussing concerns with the line manager, completing clinical incident reports and so on. Whistle blowing provides a further avenue to raise issues of concern; however, other avenues should be utilised first as appropriate.

The Public Interest Disclosure Act (1998) provides statutory protection for employees who disclose information in the public interest and are victimised because of this. The Health Service Circular 1999/198 (NHS Executive, 1999) places a responsibility on Trusts to have in place local policies and procedures which comply with the Public Interest Disclosure Act (1998). This includes the identification of a designated senior manager with responsibility to address concerns that are raised in confidence, together with a commitment that concerns raised will be investigated and taken seriously.

Protocols, procedures and clinical guidelines for quality care

Protocols, procedures and clinical guidelines are tools for ensuring quality in health-care delivery. The term procedure refers to clinical interventions that are constituted as step-by-step actions to be followed when performing a particular clinical activity. Examples of procedures include:

- Hand washing
- Intra muscular injection
- Taking physiological measurements such as blood pressure
- Mouth care/oral hygiene.

In nursing and midwifery, procedures entail taking an individualised, holistic and evidence-based approach to care, with the awareness that the skill can be performed from novice to competent, and to expert practice levels. They are expanded role activities that involve specialist training, assessment and super-vised practice.

According to Dukes and Stewart (1993), a protocol consists of recommendations, suggestions, helpful hints, or rules to be followed, requirements or standards for any medical situation where rational procedures can be specified and for use by one or more healthcare professionals in multi-disciplinary teams, and also by patients or service users and their relatives. Thus, protocols are also for use by multi-disciplinary team members, and by patients (Carroll, 1997). Dukes and Stewart (1993) note that the advantages of having protocols are that they:

- raise standards of treatment;
- improve the management of chronic disease, both by setting out best practice and by ensuring that there is seamless care by different clinicians;
- improve medical training;
- provide a means of monitoring performance;
- make preventive medicine more widely available by controlled delegation to other staff;
- make costs predictable and so improve budgeting;

- reduce costs;
- protect from litigation because a clinician can say that he or she followed the protocol for treatment;
- promote best practice;
- standardise care; and
- ensure that the standard of care given to patients/clients does not fall below a defined minimum standard.

The likely disadvantages or dangers of protocols are that they (Dukes and Stewart, 1993):

- can freeze practice on unsound treatment and inhibit the introduction of improvements. It is the frequent differences of opinion as to which is the best treatment that can make protocol writing so contentious;
- get out of date;
- make it difficult to individualise patient care;
- can restrict the use of clinical discretion or own clinical judgement;
- increase costs;
- can promote ritualistic behaviour;
- can be seen as too prescriptive; and
- may lead to overriding of the patient's rights.

The meanings of the term protocols and clinical guidelines overlap. The latter is defined by the Institute for Medicine (1992) as systematically developed statements which assist practitioners and patients to make decisions about appropriate healthcare in specific clinical circumstances. National clinical guidelines can comprise broad statements of good practice with little operational detail, and are used to inform the development of protocols. Local clinical guidelines are also referred to as protocols. Clinical guidelines available for your specialism in your organisation might include:

- Cannulation
- Defibrillation
- Suturing
- Patient group directions (PGDs)
- Drug administration
- Radiological requests by non-medical healthcare practitioners
- Wound management.

When developing a clinical guideline, the healthcare practitioner should ensure that they address the following:

- A lead clinician is identified for the clinical guideline.
- A clearly identified rationale is recorded.
- The guideline is evidence-based.
- The development process includes input from the various groups of staff that will be required to utilise the guideline.
- The guideline is ratified in accordance with the ratification process of the respective organisation.

- The guideline supports person-centred care.
- The guideline includes mechanisms for monitoring, for example, audit.
- A review date is agreed, together with the opportunity to amend prior to the review date if necessary.

Clinical guidelines can be presented as algorithms, which are informative and concise, but might not include enough breadth and depth of information. Therefore a descriptive format might be used with summary points and concluding statements. They are usually constituted through a bottom-up approach in that they are initiated and devised by specialists in the particular clinical area. The NHS Executive (1996) identified criteria that can be utilised to appraise clinical guidelines as follows:

- Valid
- Reproducible
- Reliable
- Cost-effective
- Representative
- Clinical applicability
- Flexible
- Clear
- Reviewable
- Amenable to clinical audit.

Procedures, protocols and clinical guidelines are essential resources at the disposal of the DCM for the delivery of care of a very high standard, but they need to be regularly appraised for their evidence base.

Good practice guidelines for ensuring quality in healthcare

- Monitor and review the quality performance of your practice setting in relation to identified quality metrics and compare performance against that of other practice settings within the organisation.
- Discuss quality and safety issues as part of team handover and meetings, and explore ways that quality can be further improved within your practice setting.
- As you go about your day-to-day activities, ask patients about their experiences and whether they have any suggestions regarding how care could be improved.
- Ensure a high standard of record keeping within your practice setting.
- Monitor team members' compliance with policies, procedures and guidelines.
- Complete risk assessments and document interventions to reduce the likelihood of risk occurring.
- Complete clinical incident reports to report clinical incidents and near misses.

Chapter summary

As explored within the chapter, the DCM has an important role in assuring quality in healthcare delivery and patient safety and quality of care delivery within the practice setting. Clinical Governance provides a framework for quality assurance within healthcare, the various component parts of which are explored throughout the chapters within the book. The DCM also has a key role in ensuring that the patient experience is a positive one and that customer care principles are applied within the practice setting. The DCM needs to act as a champion and role model for quality and safety and to ensure that policies, procedures and guidelines are followed and standards of care are maintained and improved upon. This chapter has therefore addressed:

- the concept quality, quality assurance and total quality management;
- some of the more practical quality assurance frameworks namely Clinical Governance, Maxwell's elements of quality and Donabedian's structure, process and outcome model, as well as the monitoring of quality in healthcare;
- patient safety and the roles of the NPSA and the WHO;
- service improvement techniques, including process mapping, metrics, 'lean', releasing time to care, root cause analysis, plan-do-study-act and benchmarking;
- the patient experience, such as patient satisfaction surveys, improving the patient experience, complaints and whistle blowing; and
- protocols and clinical guidelines for quality care, ending with good practice guidelines for ensuring quality in healthcare.

SIX Managing change, developments and innovations in practice settings

Introduction

Change is a necessary feature of all forward looking organisations. Healthcare organisations in particular are subject to ongoing change as an inevitable necessity, and for a number of unavoidable reasons, change is also ubiquitous. This chapter explores why change occur in practice settings and the DCM's role in managing changes, including initiating, participating in and influencing change.

Chapter objectives

On completion of this chapter you will be able to:

- indicate the various changes that impact on healthcare organisations and on clinical practice;
- ascertain the reasons for change in healthcare, their impact in practice settings and the significance of the management of change;
- explain how to manage change using the RAPSIES model for effective change management; and
- demonstrate how you have developed your skills in the management of change.

Changes in care and treatment

Changes in healthcare practitioners' activities are often initiated by new evidence and are usually related to ensuring quality of care, as discussed in Chapter 5, and often also driven by targets set by government reform, policy and the need to maximise outcomes for patients. Other reasons for change include new and more effective technology, research and rising consumer expectations.

 Action point 6.1 – Changes in hands-on care

Reflect on how care is currently delivered in your workplace, and identify aspects of care delivery that have changed recently?

Next, identify an aspect of practice in your work setting that you consider would benefit from change. This may be in relation to an article that you have read recently or discussion with colleagues regarding how they do things in their practice setting.

You should be able to identify several examples of changes or developments in clinical practice. Examples of such changes are identified in Box 6.1.

Box 6.1: Examples of changes affecting care delivery

- Cardio-pulmonary resuscitation (CPR) techniques
- Modified early warning score (MEWS) for critically ill patients
- Cognitive behaviour therapy for depressive illnesses
- Non-medical prescribing e.g. nurse prescribing
- Increased health education by community nurses to empower patients and enhance self-care
- Treatment of leg ulcers – using Doppler technique
- Meals served on a colour-coded tray to indicate the patient's level of ability to feed themselves
- Health MOT for all over 75s
- Non-medical practitioners ordering X-rays and other diagnostic tests
- Needle-safe devices
- Using pH indicator strips to determine location of nasogastric tube in neonates
- Zero tolerance of violent or aggressive behaviour by patients or their visitors

---

With regard to two items in Box 6.1, for instance, the new CPR guidelines changed resuscitation practice from the previous ratio of chest compressions to rescue breaths, to thirty chest compressions to two rescue breaths (Resuscitation Council, 2005). For needle safe devices, this also comprises a relatively recent development that is deliberately designed to sample blood safely, avoid needle stick injuries, prevent cross-infection and also provide extra comfort for both patient and professional (Morton Medical, 2004). Examples of recent changes in the organisation or management of care include:

- Single Assessment Process (SAP) for older people
- Introducing new shift patterns
- Integrated care pathways (ICP)
- Team midwifery and the development of the CSW role in midwifery
- Outreach work
- Quality assurance programmes, such as patient satisfaction surveys
- Allowing parents to be present in the anaesthetic room
- Intermediate care services
- NHS Direct
- Drop-in centres
- The modern matron role
- Separate facilities for men and women in mental health hospital wards.

With the SAP for older people for example, while previously several healthcare practitioners in the acute, community and social care sectors conducted assessments to identify health or social needs of older people, now only one healthcare practitioner performs the assessment and subsequent care is planned so that it is more effective and coordinated, thorough and accurate, but without procedures being needlessly duplicated by different agencies.

Changes usually occur in response to a number of drivers or catalysts, which in addition to the reasons discussed earlier in this chapter include evaluations of services, complaints and suggestions, national targets, rising expectations and competition. At times, changes occur naturally in practice settings. However, implementers of change also need to consider when the time is right for the change to be introduced, with consideration also given to other initiatives and changes that are already being implemented. Changes can be implemented at organisational or individual level in the practice setting.

Change can be differentiated from innovation in that a change occurs to something that is already established and can mean developing the clinical activity by adding extra dimensions, substituting aspects of the activity, or reverting to an older (but effective) mode of practice. Innovation relates to the introduction of a new initiative that is relatively unprecedented.

Why changes in healthcare and why the management of change?

Change is essential for improvement and modernisation of health services, to be successful the change needs to be effectively led and managed.

Why changes in healthcare?

One of the prominent reasons for the DCM requiring expertise in the management of change is that the manager's role includes change management as identified under the 'Clinician and practice developer' role in Chapter 2, and in Mintzberg's (1990) management role theory as 'entrepreneurial roles' (as noted in Chapter 2), which in turn implies innovating and implementing new ideas. Thus change is closely related to clinical practice development, which is discussed shortly.

Another reason for change is the growth of 'nurse entrepreneurs' who initiate new nursing interventions that benefit patient care, as highlighted in journal articles and reports such as by Collinson (2000) and Liefer (2005). Drennan (2007) reports on a study that explored nurse, midwife and health visitor entrepreneurship in the United Kingdom, from which she devised a typology of entrepreneurs. In the first category of the typology, she distinguished between entrepreneurs and intrapreneurs, the latter focusing on innovations and change pioneered by the organisation's own employees. The second category comprised 'infrastructure services' such as non-medical consultants, independent healthcare practitioners and inventors; and in the third category are, for instance, primary care services such as non-medical services including complementary therapists and nurse-general practitioner partners. Entrepreneurship is publicised and advocated in various DH documents such as *Our Health, Our Care, Our Say* (DH, 2006a).

Evidence-based healthcare (EBHC)

One of the key triggers for changes in care delivery is EBHC, which is defined as an approach to decision-making in which the healthcare practitioner uses the 'best evidence' available for making clinical decisions (Gray, 2001). Thus without available evidence, or the use of those that are available, practice risks becoming out of date very quickly. There are five key elements of EBHC, namely:

1 Decisions are based on best evidence.
2 Nature and sources of evidence are determined by the problem.
3 Best evidence integrates research and personal experience.
4 Evidence is translated into action so that it affects patients' or service users' health and well-being positively.
5 These actions are continually appraised.

There are differences between the overlapping terms EBHC, EBP and EBM. EBHC tends to refer to groups of patients and the management of longer-term conditions for instance, whereas EBP refers to single clinical interventions. EBM is an abbreviation for evidence-based medicine, and refers purely to medical practice rather than broader healthcare practice. Evidence-based management, evidence-based education and evidence-based assessment of competence are also well documented in the healthcare literature.

There are a number of possible sources of evidence that can support improvements in care. These include:

- Randomised controlled trials (RCT)
- Qualitative studies
- Personal experience
- Personal intuition
- Policy directives (from local sources/central/ local government legislation)
- Textbooks
- Own professional education
- Clinical guidelines
- The patient/client/family
- Colleagues/other professionals
- Trial and error
- Suppliers' information
- Journal articles
- On-line references
- Unpublished evidence
- Overview of evidence by specific topic (i.e. critical appraisals).

The Cochrane library which is accessible via the Internet or library databases at the local university, NHS Trust or National Library for Health (www.library.nhs.uk) are usually the nearest avenue for accessing published sources of evidence. The evidence available can be categorised as grades or levels of evidence to identify the strength of evidence supporting the intervention. In broad terms five levels of evidence can be identified, namely:

Level 1: Very strong evidence based on a critical appraisal of several well-designed randomised controlled trials (RCT)
Level 2: Evidence based on at least one well-designed RCT
Level 3: Evidence from several quantitative studies

Level 4:   Conclusions from one well-designed quantitative study or from qualitative studies

Level 5:   Conclusions drawn by experts in the field and in authoritative organisations

When applying evidence to practice, the patient needs to be provided with the relevant information to enable them to make an informed choice. A systematic review of randomised controlled trials may represent the 'gold standard', but this option may not be the preferred choice for the patient.

Clinical practice development

Consider the developments in clinical practice that are currently occurring in your particular area of practice, and the changes that have been made recently or can be made to specific care and treatments in your practice setting. Changes and innovations in patient related clinical practice is also known as clinical practice development. This concept therefore refers to changing the way particular clinical interventions are performed, or for providing (or installing) new healthcare services for patients. It has to do with improving and enhancing clinical practice where there is scope to do so.

The RCN (2006a:1) defines practice development as 'an approach that helps you, your team and organisation to provide care that patients feel is right for them'. This definition is a little brief and broad, and a more helpful definition is provided by Garbett and McCormack (2002:88), who suggest that:

> Practice development is a continuous process of improvement towards increased effectiveness in person-centred care. This is brought about by enabling healthcare teams to develop their knowledge and skills, and to transform the culture and context of care. It is enabled and supported by facilitators committed to a systematic, rigorous and continuous process of emancipatory change that reflect the perspectives of both service users and service providers.

Clearly the focus of the definition is on improving outcomes for patients. The term clinical practice development has to do with changes in hands-on patient care interventions for particular components of professional practice. Practice development is by no means a new phenomenon, as healthcare practitioners have always looked out for ways of delivering safer and more effective care and treatment for patients.

The DCM needs to take an analytical approach to the development of practice; which can be achieved in various ways. Based on an analysis of literature, focus group interviews with practice developers and individual interviews with healthcare practitioners on practice development, Garbett and McCormack (2002) conclude that the purpose of practice development is to increase effectiveness in patient-centred care, and transform care and the culture and context within which it takes place. The attributes of practice development are that it needs to be systematic and rigorous, a continuous process, and founded on facilitation. The consequences of practice development include improved experiences of care in terms of their sensitivity to the needs of individuals and populations for users; and increased capacity of autonomous practice for practitioners. The four main themes that emerged from the study were that (p. 92):

1 it is a means of improving patient care;
2 it transforms the contexts and cultures in which healthcare delivery takes place;
3 it ensures that a systematic approach is employed to effect changes in practice; and
4 various types of facilitation are required for change to take place.

Identifying the purposes, attributes and consequences of practice development constitutes an exercise that ensures a cautious and planned approach to change. Concluding from a four-year action research study related to a task-centred service to a patient-centred service, Titchen (2003) identifies three generic principles of practice development which she suggests comprises a conceptual framework. These principles are:

1 Changing the practice philosophy
2 Putting the process of change into practice
3 Investing in practice development.

McCormack et al. (2006) report on a study that indicates that practice development comprises of six crucial components, namely: policy and strategy, methodology and methods, roles and relationships, learning strategies, funding and evaluating effectiveness. How the DCM achieves such change will be discussed under how to manage change later in this chapter. Furthermore, practice development can be undertaken at individual level, particularly by those who have autonomy in their day-to-day work; at unit or team level; or at organisational or supra-organisational levels. The Donabedian (1988) model of evaluation, which comprises considering and identifying the standard to be achieved, along with structure, process and outcome is a systematic approach that can be adopted to monitor the effectiveness of the development.

Structure refers to the equipment, staff and materials required; process refers to the procedure, training and ongoing evaluation of the activity; and outcome refers to the exact final product. In the context of practice development, structure or approach refers to identifying the practice development function as part of annual IDPR for instance. As to process or deployment, for some staff such as practice development nurses, this comprises the main focus of their role. However, each team member can be a practice developer and this is evident in the *NHS KSF* (DH, 2004a) under the 'service improvement' domain.

Another very influential organisation constantly innovating healthcare is the NHS Institute of Innovation and Improvement (NHS III) (2007a, b), which took over much of the work previously being done by the NHS Modernisation Agency. This organisation supports the NHS to transform healthcare for patients and the public by rapidly developing and disseminating new ways of working, new technology and leadership, in, for example:

• improving care for people with long-term conditions;
• mental health;
• cancer care;

- stroke;
- hospital waiting: the 18-week patient pathway; and
- guiding and helping leaders to reduce avoidable deaths.

Some of the key publications on practice enhancement include RCN and DH's (RCN, 2005b) *Maxi nurses: Nurses Working in Advanced and Extended Roles Promoting and Developing Patient-centred Healthcare*, and DH (2002) *Liberating the Talents: Helping Primary Care Trusts and Nurses to Deliver the NHS Plan*.

Why 'manage' change?

Change is essential within healthcare to ensure that care is based on the best available evidence, new technology is embraced and that the available resources are maximised. Change can:

- be imposed;
- be introduced after brief discussions;
- evolve gradually over time;
- be self-directed, such as in lifestyle or behaviour change; and
- be managed.

Change, needs to be 'managed' if it is to be successfully implemented and sustained.

 Action point 6.2 – Ways of making changes

Consider a recent change in your practice setting and think about the way the change was made, taking into account the five categories of change identified above.

Change can have different effects on different individuals such as:

1 stress;
2 excitement;
3 involvement and ownership;
4 will have gained more individual responsibility; and
5 will improve patient care.

How to manage change

The management of change involves taking a planned and systematic approach. One such approach can be the '7-step RAPSIES model for effective change management' (see Figure 6.1). This model is derived from the extensive literature on the topic and on our own experience as healthcare practitioners. The 7-step model comprises the

Figure 6.1 *The RAPSIES framework for effective change management*

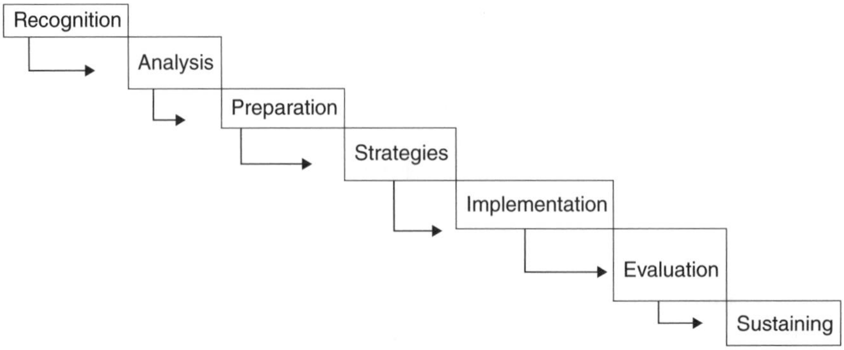

essential components of the management of change, which are as follows:

1 **Recognition** of the need for change to solve a problem for instance, or to improve an element of practice.
2 **Analysis** of the available options related to the contemplated change, the environment or setting where change will be implemented and the users of the change.
3 **Preparation** for the change, such as identifying a change agent to lead the implementation of the change, education, defining intended outcomes and involving relevant colleagues.
4 **Strategies** for implementing the change (explained later in this chapter).
5 **Implementation** of the change including piloting the change and timing of implementation.
6 **Evaluation** of the impact of the change against the intended outcomes.
7 **Sustaining** the change, i.e. how to ensure the change endures and is mainstreamed.

Recognising the need for change

Staff dissatisfaction with the way care is delivered, complaints received from patients or their relatives, and new research findings on how to improve care are some of the factors that indicate the need for change. Several other reasons were identified earlier in this chapter under 'why changes in healthcare?' One of the most significant attributes of change is that it must represent relative advantage over the status quo, in that it must benefit the patient and/or the organisation through an improvement in outcomes. For example, if changing to using a new scientifically tested care package, this should improve patient care, and have specific benefits in terms of patient outcomes.

The change must also be compatible with the team's existing beliefs and values about healthcare delivery at a philosophical as well as pragmatic level. How easily it can be understood by patients and stakeholders must also be considered. The simplicity or the ease of using the change or innovation, and its trialability, that is, the possibility of piloting the innovation must also be considered, as well as observability, that is, the change and its results must be tangible.

Analysis of the change

After identifying that a change is needed, the healthcare practitioner needs to explore all options available before deciding on the best solution. For instance, in relation to the issue of ensuring that in-patients receive adequate nutrition, you may identify a number of changes to achieve this, such as:

- reducing other activities during meal times;
- implementing snack trolleys;
- staggering meal times;
- implementing volunteer feeders;
- implementing a 'red tray' system;
- asking for feedback on the quality of meals;
- implementing protected meal times; and
- ensuring assistance with eating is given to those who need it.

Several examples of real-life changes in healthcare delivery implemented by healthcare practitioners can be cited, such as using the most appropriate dressings on particular wounds, and implementing a redesigned sedation scoring system for critically ill patients in intensive care units. The DH (2006a) for instance cites several other examples, such as peer-mentoring introduced by school nurses and NHS 'Life Check' service. In response to Action point 6.1, you should have been able to identify a number of examples of changes in care delivery in your area of practice.

On deciding which specific change(s) is to be made, those involved need to consider the advantages and likely disadvantages of the change. This comprises an analysis of the specific change in more systematic ways such as by force field or SWOT analyses that are discussed shortly.

The users of the change

Analysis of the proposed change includes careful consideration of the users of the change. Planning includes selling the change to the users, and exploring developmental needs as individuals or as a team. Rogers and Shoemaker (1971) identified six categories of users of change:

1	Innovators	– Individuals in the team who get excited about new ideas and are keen to implement them
2	Early adopters	– Individual team members who think about the new change over a few days and then adopt them
3	Early majority	– When a few team members adopt the new idea
4	Later majority	– When several members accept and adopt the new idea
5	Laggards	– Individuals who tend to lag behind in adopting new ways of working
6	Rejecters	– Individuals who are against new ideas or usually oppose them

Action point 6.3 – The users of change in my practice setting

Consider your work colleagues and their response to a recent change that has been implemented in your practice setting. See if you can identify those who could fall into each of the categories identified by Rogers and Shoemaker. Suggest ways in which you could use the information about users of change to support the change management process.

With innovators, the change agent can for instance use their energy and allocate them responsibilities. The remaining categories of users comprise those who resist change either momentarily or longer term. Early adopters need recognition for their compliance with the change, whereas those who form the later majority are individuals who need more time to assimilate the new concept, to try it out and use the change. Laggards may need extra support and time to prevent disillusionment. As for rejecters, the change agent or the line manager will need to explore further to identify possible reasons for this. The employee, may for example, be experiencing transient personal problems, or be privy to further knowledge in relation to the change.

The setting or environment where the change is to be implemented

Another essential component of change management is the setting or environment where the change is to be implemented. The environment has to be 'ripe for change' for successful implementation. A clinical environment that is conducive to change manifests:

- a progressive ethos where critical appraisal, creativity and openness are fostered;
- good channels of communication, that is, two-way and effective communication that include opportunities for feedback and evaluation;
- a cohesive team who work in partnership with the patient as the focus;
- team empowerment, that is, the freedom to be innovative and creative within the wider organisation; and
- supportive leadership that actively promotes and supports a 'can do' approach.

From the critical analysis viewpoint, some of the factors that constitute barriers to research implementation or utilisation include:

- Palfreyman et al.'s (2003) findings that nurses and physiotherapists have access to a wide variety of sources of knowledge, but both professions have problems overcoming the barrier of time.
- '… important research findings are not having the desired impact on practice' (West et al., 1999:633).
- '… dissemination failings represent the single most significant factor in the research-practice gap' (Dickson, 1996:5).

Action point 6.4 – Current relevance of Hunt's findings

Consider the current relevance of Hunt's (1997) suggestions regarding barriers to research and whether they still apply today. Do you feel they do?

Other barriers to research implementation faced by clinicians that are suggested by Professor Hunt (1997) are:

- lack of critical appraisal and research skills;
- lack of time to undertake research;
- not having access to the right resources;
- an organisational and managerial ethos and culture expecting instant answers;
- lack of power and financial control to make things happen; and
- lack of valid research on any one topic, or of user friendly reviews and guidelines.

McCaughan (2002) suggests that barriers to research implementation include:

1 problems in interpreting and using research – it is seen as too complex, 'academic' and overly statistical;
2 even healthcare practitioners who feel confident with research-based information experience a lack of organisational support;
3 researchers and findings lack clinical credibility and fail to offer sufficient clinical direction; and
4 some healthcare practitioners lack the skills and motivation to use research themselves.

Preparation for change

The change agent

The DCM's role in implementing change involves being both a change agent and a supporter of changes that are being implemented. Alternatively, the change agent could be a facilitator external to the organisation, or an employee within the organisation, the department or the practice setting itself. The change agent is the person who is assigned to advocate, lead and implement the change, and might also be the initiator of the change. They need to be completely clear about the present state of readiness in the setting, and the potential future state after the change has been implemented.

In considering 'readiness for change' the change agent needs to consider how adequately staffed the area is to accommodate the change or new practice. Human resource issues therefore need to be addressed, but the change agent must also be cognisant of the components of change in the seven-steps to effective change management, which of course includes sustaining the change after implementation. The change agent's key functions include:

- selling the change and promoting ownership by the clinical team;
- planning the change comprehensively;
- determining and deciding on relevant change strategies;

- identifying own and others' related development needs;
- monitoring and supporting the change users throughout the process;
- evaluating the impact of the change;
- problem-solving to address any challenges that are experienced; and
- sustaining the change.

The characteristics of an effective change agent are also those of being an effective leader. Two leadership styles that are particularly relevant for managing change are transformational and transactional styles. The transactional style refers to the orderly breaking down of tasks but the transformational style constitutes keeping a distance, and taking a strategic or 'helicopter' view of the whole. Table 3.1 in Chapter 3 identifies some of the characteristics of the two styles of leadership.

The change agent's role thus incorporates dissemination of the evidence or knowledge base, on which change is being advocated and initiated. Scullion (2002) suggests that dissemination is a vital yet complex process that aims to ensure that key messages are conveyed to specific groups via a wide range of methods so that it results in some reaction, some impact or implementation. Methods of research dissemination include:

- Via professional associations
- Video/DVD/audio tape
- Written reports as feedback to respondents/research subjects
- Written executive summaries (most likely to be read if concise)
- Books, or chapters in books
- Journal articles or editorials
- Journal clubs
- Conferences
- Poster presentation
- Newsletters
- Inclusion in course curriculum
- Educational materials.

As for the users of the change, which can include your colleagues or patients, the key factors in the dissemination process include consideration of how ready they are to use the change, enabling them to become active agents for the change, rather than passive recipients, forming social networks, and choosing suitable strategies for that particular group of users.

Furthermore, change can evoke anxiety, and resistance to change can prevail because of:

- fear of the unknown;
- lack of confidence;
- lack of knowledge and skills to carry out the change;
- loss of influence and power; and
- resentment of perceived criticism of past practices.

For each of these components causing resistance to change, the DCM or change agent can take specific actions to manage them. For 'fear of the unknown', this presents a degree of uncertainty, and the change agent for instance can provide detailed and sufficient information to those who are resisting the change so that they become fully familiar with the proposed change. For lack of confidence, further information and support can be provided. For lack of knowledge and skills to carry out the change, organising workshops and study days might prove beneficial. For loss of influence and power, the key tasks can be made more explicit. For resentment of perceived criticism of past practices, the attributes of the change should be highlighted or emphasised as progressing to further improvements in care.

In addition, people get accustomed to established practices as they feel comfortable and secure with them. They might also resist if they feel overburdened by too much change at a point in time, or if they feel the change is likely to reduce freedom or result in increased control of their movements; increased work at the same level of pay; people feel more secure in using well-established ways, and wish to retain old ways of practice. Therefore, the need for change should emerge through a bottom-up approach including active involvement in planning, implementation and evaluation of the process.

Strategies for implementing change

The discussion so far indicates that change needs to be managed, it needs to be planned thoroughly and it needs to be participative to promote ownership. Various strategies are documented in the management literature that can be selected according to their suitability for a particular change and practice setting. Strategies for effective organisational change will now be critiqued and include:

- Plan-do-study-act
- Lewin's three-stage process
- Empirical-rational
- Power-coercive
- Normative-re-educative

Plan-do-study-act

The PDSA cycle (IHI, 2007) (see Figure 6.2) comprises a strategy for testing the impact of an identified change within the work setting. It allows testing to be undertaken on a small scale with the opportunity to refine it prior to its wider application.

Figure 6.2 *Plan-do-study-act cycle*

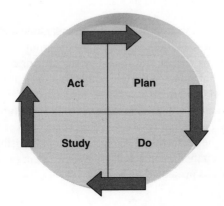

Action point 6.5 – Implementing change

Think about a change that you would like to implement within your clinical area/ service. In order to support you to test the change, develop a PDSA cycle that addresses the following areas that have been adapted from the IHI model:

Plan
- What you are hoping to achieve
- What you think the outcome of the change will be
- The support you consider you will need to be able to implement the change
- The mechanisms you intend to use to test the impact of the change

Do
- Implement the change in the identified area
- Observe the change and document any problems that are encountered
- Commence analysis of the data that you have collected

Study
- Complete the data analysis
- Compare the results achieved with those that you predicted in the planning phase
- Summarise and reflect upon what you have learnt

Act
- Using what you have learnt from the test, identify any modifications that you need to make
- Prepare your plan of action for the next test

Lewin's three-stage process of change

A programme of planned change and improved performance developed by Lewin (1951) involves a three-stage process entailing unfreezing, movement and refreezing.

Unfreezing – refers to reducing those forces which maintain behaviour in its present form and recognition of the need for change and improvement to occur.

Movement – refers to the development of new attitudes or behaviours and the implementation of the change.

Refreezing – refers to stabilising the change at a new level and reinforcement through supporting mechanisms such as policies, resources and norms.

Systematic ways of unfreezing a set of circumstances include the well-known SWOT analysis, and also force field analysis, which entails the group together identifying the factors that are driving the change and those that are causing resistance. An example of a SWOT analysis for introducing flexible family friendly shifts in a practice setting for instance is presented in Figure 6.3.

Strengths and weaknesses are internal factors, while opportunities and threats are usually external to the individual or team. A SWOT analysis can be very subjective and therefore needs to be performed as a team whenever possible. Alternatively the change agent could facilitate the force field analysis, an example of which in relation to implementing an ICP is presented in Box 6.2.

Figure 6.3   *SWOT analysis: introducing flexible family friendly shifts*

STRENGTHS	WEAKNESSES
• Happier staff • Better staff retention • Encourage recruitment • Staff morale • Maximum use of staff time • Gives individual staff more time at home • Not working too many shifts for long stretches • Less stress of travelling …	• Difficult to accommodate everyone's requirements • Staff without school age children might get less annual leave in summer • Lack of communication as they may not be present at handovers • Not feeling part of the team • Poor long-term continuity • Difficulty covering annual leave, sickness
OPPORTUNITIES	THREATS
• Extra day at home for study/education • Spend more time with family • Individual can pursue other interests • Comply with 'Improving Working Lives' (DH, 2000b) guidelines	• Staff with no family might feel disadvantaged • Whether this can be legitimately explored at recruitment interviews • Tiredness • Sickness rate can go up • Some staff might be against the changes • Fitting in with practical routine

Box 6.2: Forcefield analysis of 'integrated care pathways'

Driving forces	*Resisting forces*
• Continuity of care needed • Consistent with government policy related to patient journeys • Greater patient satisfaction • Learners get fuller picture of broader influences on personal health • More opportunity for health promotion • More collaboration within MDT • Enhances patient care • Increases cost-effectiveness through patient compliance	• Staff not knowledgeable about how ICPs work • Perceived criticism of current method of care delivery • Extra paperwork • Extra staff time required, and therefore costs • Social care and healthcare funding disjunction • More resources required in terms of staff time • Too many people disseminating information • Funding • Patient information overload

The forcefield analysis in Box 6.2 has shown that many forces may be involved in driving or resisting change. According to Lewin's (1951) force field analysis theory, behaviour in any institutional setting is not static in nature, and instead it comprises a dynamic balance of socio-psychological forces working in opposite directions within the institution. The force field analysis exercise can be undertaken by a team of staff or individually to identify the factors (i.e. people, resources and systems) that might facilitate or hinder change, and by so doing it 'unfreezes' the forces that maintain behaviour in its present form.

In attempting to change a situation to a new level, after unfreezing, three enabling actions are possible: (i) increase the driving forces by adding new ones or strengthening existing ones; (ii) reduce or remove the resisting forces; or (iii) translate one or more restraining forces into driving ones. If a change agent uses say only the first of these three actions, then change may occur, but it is often unstable and quickly reverts to the original condition. A combination of all three strategies is the most effectual.

Empirical-rational

This strategy is based on the belief that people are guided by reason, that they are essentially rational, and that if they can be helped to understand the nature and reasons for the proposed change, then they are more likely to accept it. Thus, this strategy is based on empowerment through giving knowledge. Government health warnings are at times based on this strategy.

Power-coercive

The power-coercive strategy emphasises a different kind of power, that is, that based on threats of sanctions, economic or status-wise if the desired changes are not adopted, and where necessary the use of moral power, playing on feelings of guilt and shame are used.

The assumption is that those in control of the organisation will identify the need for change, and people with less power will always comply with their plans. If an empirical-rational approach does not prove as productive, then the power-coercive strategy might be used. It can include application of legitimate power to influence and secure compliance and can incorporate legal considerations.

Normative-re-educative

Individuals, groups and organisations are seen as inherently active in ascertaining how similar they are in their practices and norms to other entities. This strategy includes suggesting that the proposed change is a normal practice in other similar settings, making reference to local socio-cultural value systems, norms and attitudes, and educating users in the value and benefits of the change. It incorporates the facility for personal growth and self-actualisation.

Combined strategies

Each of the above three strategies is based on different assumptions about what makes people change or alter their behaviour and result in achievement of different degrees of success. The strategy used is chosen according to different situations, and requires that the individual or the group should be capable of, and willing to change. It also takes into account the social, political and economic factors that influence the role of the healthcare practitioner.

However, a combined strategy can be utilised that harnesses and coordinates elements of the three above strategies, but must encompass:

- rational (or validated) information;
- two-way communication and expertise in group processes;
- consensus on new norms and sanctions associated with a proposed change; and
- legitimate authority of the change agent and the power to carry it through.

The combination could be staged in that one of the three strategies might be more appropriate at the very early stages of implementation of a particular change, and another at another stage.

Implementing the change

 Action point 6.6 – Implementing the change

Consider a change that you feel would be beneficial to implement in your practice setting. Identify a comprehensive set of activities that would ensure that the change is successfully implemented and maintained. This can take the form of a detailed action plan.

The activities you have identified for successful implementation of change might include:

- plan the change thoroughly;
- attempt to create an environment conducive to change by encouraging a culture that encourages questioning, using initiative and a reflective-evaluative approach to clinical practice;
- provide means for the acquisition of knowledge and skills, feedback and support;
- identify problems, for example, resistance and barriers and build into your plan ways to overcome them;
- provide a medium for staff to share experiences;
- provide supportive leadership by being involved throughout;
- provision for evaluation and feedback so that successes and difficulties can be shared and learned from;
- encourage active participation;
- ensure that there are good channels of communication; and
- ascertain opportunities for refinement based on evaluation.

Timing of implementation

The change agent also needs to identify the most suitable implementation date for the change. This ideally needs to be the time when the users are ready and the setting is 'ripe for change'. Times to avoid include periods when more staff are on annual leave, when there are staff vacancies or long-term sickness, or when other major managerial changes are imminent, or if there is organisational resistance to the change. It also includes a time when there is openness and trust amongst staff, and morale is good.

Evaluating the change

After the change has been implemented its impact needs to be monitored both informally and in more structured ways. Informally, evaluation information can be obtained by general impressions and casual questioning. More structured ways of evaluation can involve the use of a framework, or model, of evaluation. It can be done formatively, that is, at interim intervals rather than end stages, but summatively evaluation also needs to be conducted at specific pre-determined points when the full impact of the change can be gauged.

Evaluation of the change can involve comparing outcomes to those anticipated before implementation of the change, with specific indicators such as length of hospital stay, reduction in costs and improved patient satisfaction.

Sustaining the change

After implementation, the change needs to be sustained through explicit recognition from more senior managers, and supported by the necessary resources, human and non-human. The PDSA (IHI, 2007) method can be used to test out progress on a small scale. The users of the change should be able to sense the benefits of the change after implementation.

A strategy for sustaining change should have been established at the very beginning of the implementation of the change. The term sustaining is used to signify keeping the change in good health, that is, functioning, but more importantly, developing. This requires various forms of resources, the categories of which are discussed in Chapter 7, and include:

- appropriate human resources;
- appropriate financial resources;
- monitoring mechanisms, such as regular concurrent and retrospective audits (built-in evaluation/research);
- planned evaluation of the effects or impact of the change;
- continuing skill development in the context of new equipment and devices becoming available;
- disseminating the change to obtain external views;
- users retaining ownership of the change (active user participation);
- maintaining team spirit (as discussed in Chapter 10);
- leadership of senior staff in using the change; and
- effective communication.

At times, organisational resistance to implementing or sustaining change can be experienced, which is also referred to as barriers to change. Some of the organisational barriers to change are:

- lack of understanding of the change required in role, practices, relationships;
- lack of the knowledge and skills necessary to use the new practice;

- shortage of staff;
- lack of time;
- lack of support within the management hierarchy;
- failure of the leader to identify problems;
- lack of materials/equipment to practice the new method; and
- failure of the leader to adequately plan the management of the change.

Such resistance is less apparent in organisations that reflect the characteristics of an 'effective organisation', as suggested by Beckhard and Harris (1987). These characteristics include:

- having a strategic view;
- energising others lower in the system;
- having relatively open communication;
- rewarding collaboration;
- managing conflict, not suppressing it;
- valuing difference; and
- actively learning, through feedback.

The characteristics of an effective organisation should support change management. A change endeavour can succeed or fail depending on the various factors discussed above. However, if the components of the RAPSIES framework discussed in this chapter are fully considered, then the change should be achieved as desired.

Guidelines for effective change management

The essential activities required for successful change management are as follows:

- Ensure compatibility with existing values and practices.
- Ensure users see advantages in the innovations over existing practices.
- Have detailed knowledge of various change strategies.
- Plan well in advance, and in detail.
- Analyse existing/new structures.
- Examine adaptability to the innovation.
- Assess the readiness to change.
- Ensure effective communication at all stages.
- Institute education and training at key stages.
- Recognise early adopters' efforts explicitly.
- Assess your own knowledge continuously, and update and upskill as appropriate.
- Exercise leadership skills.
- Support the change during all stages of the process.
- Encourage active participation by intended users of the change.
- Build in evaluation/research.

Chapter summary

This chapter has focused broadly on the what, why, when and how to manage change and on the DCM's role in the management of change and innovation in the practice setting, and having completed this chapter you will have explored:

- actual and potential instances of changes made in clinical practice, that is, patient-care interventions, and in the management or organisation of care;
- why changes are necessary in healthcare and the importance of effective management of change;
- how to manage change, using the RAPSIES model for effective change management', which comprises recognising the need for the change, analysis of the available options, preparation for the change, identifying strategies for implementing the change, implementation of the change, evaluating its impact and sustaining the change; and
- analysis of issues related to the management of change in practice settings, concluding with guidelines for effective change management.

SEVEN Managing resources for healthcare delivery

Introduction

The importance of effective resource management in healthcare cannot be overestimated, as without resources there would be no health service, and conversely, only a certain proportion of national income can be allocated to health services, the remainder being required for several other social provisions. A wide range of resources are required for effective healthcare delivery, and DCMs have a responsibility to use the available resources efficiently.

Chapter objectives

On completion of this chapter you will be able to:

- ascertain the specific resources required for effective healthcare delivery, and how available human and non-human resources can be used efficiently;
- analyse how various components of human resources can be managed, and the healthcare practitioner's accountability and responsibility in doing so;
- explore budget management, taking into account what budgeting is, and why and how to budget at the practice setting level in order to maximise the use of these resources; and
- ascertain the management of a range of other non-human resources such as equipment and consumables that are required for effective healthcare delivery.

Resources required for effective healthcare delivery

An extensive range of resources are required to deliver healthcare services. The NHS delivers healthcare to a total population of 57 million within the United Kingdom. For the year 2006–07 the total expenditure on health in the United Kingdom was £96 billion (HM Treasury, 2007). The projected budget for 2007–08 was £104 billion, out of a total public expenditure of just under £600 billion for the United Kingdom, which represents around 17 per cent of the total annual expenditure that is a spending of approximately £1600 on healthcare per person each year. With 1.3 million employees the NHS is also one of the biggest employers in Europe.

Health services are provided mainly through the NHS, which aims to (DH, 2007g):

- promote health and prevent ill health;
- diagnose and treat injury and disease; and
- care for those with long-term illnesses and disability who require NHS services.

There are ten Strategic Health Authorities (SHAs) in England (with parallel arrangements in Scotland, Wales and Northern Ireland), and their role is to act as the local headquarters for the NHS. These organisations were set up initially in 2002 to develop plans for improving health services in their local area, and to monitor the performance of their local NHS organisations. SHAs do not deliver NHS services, but provide leadership, coordination and support to the NHS across a defined geographical area (see Figure 7.1). SHAs lead on strategic development of the local health service and manage the performance of for instance NHS acute trusts, ambulance trusts and primary care trusts (PCT).

SHAs endeavour to look for the best way to use the resources available to deliver and improve local healthcare. This includes plans to recruit, retain and develop all NHS staff with the full range of skills that are necessary to meet service needs. SHAs have three main tasks (DH, 2007g):

- to develop a strategic framework for the health and social care community, which clarifies priorities for action in the short, medium and long term;
- to manage and improve performance, establishing performance agreements with all local NHS organisations and working to redesign care processes with a very strong focus on patient pathways; and
- to build capacity and capability in terms of people, facilities and buildings within and across organisations.

PCTs are at the centre of the NHS and their role is to make sure that all other health services are provided, including hospitals, dentists, opticians, mental health services, NHS walk-in centres, NHS Direct, patient transport (including accident and emergency), population screening, and pharmacies. They are also responsible for

Figure 7.1 *SHAs and PCTs*

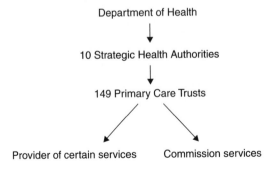

getting health and social care systems working together for the benefit of patients. The three main functions of a PCT are:

1 engaging with its local population to improve health and well-being;
2 commissioning a comprehensive and equitable range of high quality, responsive and efficient services, within allocated resources, across all service sectors; and
3 directly providing high quality responsive and efficient services where this gives best-value.

Thus PCTs have a commissioning role as well as that of a direct provider of services. They commission services for the population of an identified geographical area, and they provide services such as audiology, district nursing, health promotion, psychology services, sexual health services and wheelchair services from various locations.

The health of the nation and healthcare has featured prominently in the priorities for the various governments who have been in office. Numerous short and long-term strategies for specific aspects of healthcare are issued periodically by the DH, such as The *NHS Plan* (DH, 2000a). The March 2000 budget established that the NHS would grow by one-half in cash terms and by one-third in real terms in just five years. This strategy comprised a substantial increase in resources which included various specific targets for the NHS up to the year 2010, such as:

* 7,000 extra beds in hospitals and intermediate care
* Over 100 new hospitals by 2010 and 500 new one-stop primary care centres
* Over 3,000 GP premises modernised and 250 new scanners
* Clean wards – overseen by 'modern matrons' – and better hospital food
* Modern IT systems in every hospital and GP surgery … and investment in staff:
   – 7,500 more medical consultants and 2,000 more GPs
   – 20,000 extra nurses and 6,500 extra therapists
* 1,000 more medical school places
* Childcare support for NHS staff with 100 on-site nurseries.

Updates on progress regarding achievement of the targets of the ten-year strategy are issued principally through the DH website on various aspects of the NHS. However, it is unclear how far each of these targets has been achieved, especially with the shift from target orientation to standards and local services orientation (DH, 2006b).

A recent major landmark is the provision for healthcare trusts to apply for NHS Foundation Trust status (DH, 2007d). The basis for NHS Foundation Trusts is that it devolves decision-making from central Government to local healthcare organisations such as acute, specialist and mental health hospitals. Nonetheless, as noted in Chapter 1, a further review of NHS services and resourcing started in July 2007, and the findings and recommendations were published in June 2008 (DH, 2008a).

Each healthcare trust is a separate organisation, and each NHS healthcare trust is ultimately managed by a chairman and their Board, with a Chief Executive appointed for general management. The Chief Executive's remit is to ensure appropriate structures are instituted so that operational activities achieve the aims of the trust. These aims, along with the trust's mission statement and objectives are stated in the operational (usually annual), and strategic (usually five to ten years) plans. These documents state the vision for the future for the organisation. Subsequently, business plans are also determined with further specific details, including the resources required for meeting particular strategic aims.

Decisions made at trust's Board meetings impact directly on DCMs' roles in delivering the services that are supported, and human and material resources are made available for them. Regular budget statements are issued to indicate areas of underspend and overspend to enable budget holders to monitor their expenditure. The next section considers all of the resources that are required for delivering care in practice settings.

Resources at ward/unit/department/trust level

As noted earlier, various resources are required for an organisation to function effectively and appropriate resources are required in practice settings to support the delivery of healthcare.

 Action point 7.1 – Resources for healthcare trusts

List all of the resources that the DCM requires in the day-to-day management of the practice setting.

As the word resource signifies, it constitutes items and means that enable the achievement of organisation goals. In response to the above action point you might have mentioned that the resources required for most practice settings include staff and money for staff salaries, and for purchasing, maintaining and repairing equipment and so on. Organisations generally differentiate between human resources (or pay expenses) and non-human resources (or non-pay expenses or consumables). Another classification comprises grouping resources under human and hardware resources, namely:

Human resources: For example, staff's clinical knowledge, their skills and time.
Hardware resources: For example, accommodation, medications, equipment.

A wide range of human and non-human resources need to be available for the management of healthcare delivery. They can be grouped under the acronym BEICHMM, which stands for:

- Buildings
- Equipments
- Information technology
- Consumables
- Human resources
- Methods
- Money.

BEICHMM comprises a framework that can be used to determine all of the resources required by the organisation or by the practice setting. The need for one main building or a number of *buildings* is obviously necessary to accommodate the designated healthcare delivery facilities. *Equipment* as resources includes X-ray machines, telephones, manual handing aids, patient attached equipment such as cardiac monitors or syringe drivers, specialist equipment that is pertinent to the area, for example, a minibus for use by patients within a rehabilitation service. For *consumables*, the resources comprise disposable single-use items.

Human resources, or workforce, refers to all categories of staff (e.g. nursing, AHPs, medical staff, CSWs, ancillary staff, managers and administrators, etc.), and therefore include the correct skill mix of staff (qualified and unqualified, specialists, etc.), communications, recruitment and retention. It includes consideration of pending maternity leave and retirement, which creates temporary or longer-term vacancies. It also includes having to make a case for more staff, contingency requirements, for example, if there is an increase in the number of influenza sufferers during winter months, and the training, continued professional development (CPD) and motivation of staff.

Methods as resources include procedures, policies, protocols and clinical procedures, together with the training to be able to use them. It includes ways of meeting professional updating requirements for structuring of care by ICPs for instance, and for making referrals to medical staff, specialist nurses and therapists. For *money*, the resources include the cost of maintaining the building(s), equipment, the cost of employing staff and so on; in short, all other resources just mentioned.

Healthcare resources need to be utilised efficiently. Efficiency refers to the achievement of expected objectives at minimum financial cost, in the minimum amount of time, but to the required standard. It refers to achieving maximum effect from available resources. The associated term effectiveness refers to the appropriateness and extent of what is being achieved and should be measurable in terms of patient outcomes.

Managers are accountable for the efficient use of the money allocated to the trust, and they have to manage all resources responsibly. Resourcing care and treatment in hospitals and primary care settings is challenging as novel treatment methods and new medications for conditions that have thus far proved difficult to manage appear and compete for a proportion of the NHS budget.

It is important to note therefore that the health service is a cash-limited service and therefore the decisions made regarding the allocation of resources are critical. There can also be challenges faced in the management of resources, for example, delays experienced in the appointment of staff, and receiving requirement equipment, or servicing those already in use, together with depreciation and replacement costs.

Why 'manage' resources?

There are several reasons why the DCM needs to be knowledgeable about how resources are managed. Cash-limited financial resources allocated to the NHS are predominantly taxpayers' money, and therefore need to be managed intelligently and responsibly.

How resources are utilised needs careful planning, which means deciding in advance the activities that the trust plans to engage in, how they will be achieved and which personnel will ensure they are. It involves considering economy, effectiveness and efficiency in the use of resources, and the accountability and responsibility of resource managers.

The remainder of this chapter discusses the management of healthcare resources in two major parts: human resources, which include skill mix, recruitment and retention of staff, and expectations from each other by the organisation and its staff; and non-human resources, namely budgets, equipment, information technology, consumables as well as protocols and guidelines for care delivery.

Managing human resources

With his notion of 'upside down thinking', Handy (1984) is well-known for suggesting that employees should be treated as assets rather than costs, and hence investing in them. Armstrong (2006) suggests that employees should be perceived as 'human capital', implying they should be treated as assets that the organisations value. If this logic is followed, then in health services employees should be treated as their most valuable resources, who should be managed in appropriate ways to enable them to fulfil their roles in a way that is mutually beneficial.

The concept of human resource management (HRM) has evolved over the last few decades from referring to the employees of the organisation as workers who cost money in terms of wages that are paid to them, to recognising them as individuals who contribute to the success of the organisation. It is defined by Armstrong (2006:3) as 'a strategic and coherent approach to the management of an organisation's most valued assets – the people working there who individually and collectively contribute to the achievement of the objectives of the business'.

Mullins (2007:805) suggests that HRM is the 'design, implementation and maintenance of strategies to manage people for optimum business performance including the development of policies and processes to support these strategies'. HRM, therefore, aims to improve the productive contribution of individual employees whilst simultaneously attempting to attain the employer's, societal and individual employee's objectives.

In healthcare, HRM largely refers to ensuring that appropriate individuals are employed with the right skills and in right numbers at the time to ensure that the healthcare organisation's goals are achieved. As a management technique, HRM endeavours to ensure that employees are appointed to the right places, in the right jobs and at the right times.

 Action point 7.2 – Specific human resources in healthcare

Identify as many particular categories of staff who contribute to healthcare delivery as you can in your healthcare organisation.

An appropriate range of resources are required to ensure organisations achieve their annual and long-term aims and objectives. Grouped under human and non-human resources, the former refers to all employees, namely:

- Managers at various levels
- Administrative staff
- Estates department employees – such as those who maintain the site, buildings and so on
- Medical practitioners – including consultants and junior doctors
- Nurses, midwives and CSWs
- Allied health professionals
- Ancillary staff – porters, electricians, plumbers
- Catering staff
- Pathology staff and laboratory technicians
- Chaplains/faith representatives
- Gardeners
- Housekeepers.

Skill mix

Naturally, the various personnel identified in response to Action point 7.2 are crucial for effective treatment and care delivery. This comprises an appropriate combination of qualified healthcare practitioners and unqualified staff who are trained and competent in selected skills. This combination is referred to as skill mix, which is a term that refers to the numbers and ratio, capability and experience of qualified and unqualified staff.

On examining the tools available for the systematic assessment of skill mix, Hurst (2006) concludes that there are some quick and easy methods as well as those that are more complex. The three main methods utilised are (i) the top-down method used by workforce planners, (ii) professional judgement methods based on consensus with colleagues and (iii) bottom-up methods which are workload driven, and based on patient demands at clinical level. Hurst identifies various categories of bottom-up methods, but notes that there is no perfect method as each has strengths and weaknesses. The Healthcare Commission (2005) reports however that nurse staffing methods are predominantly unsystematic and irrational.

Earlier methods of gauging skill mix were criticised for being aimed at reducing the ratio of qualified to unqualified staff, and for shifting workload on to CSWs. It included so-called 'unproductive time' that is, paid meal breaks and rest periods, and discussion on subjects not related to work.

The reason for ensuring the correct skill mix in practice settings is that various studies (e.g. RCN, 2006b; Rafferty et al., 2007) support the argument that quality of care improves proportionately to the number of more qualified staff available, and patient outcomes are better when nurses care for fewer patients. Such studies indicate that a poor skill mix of qualified and unqualified nurses lead to comparatively poorer patient outcomes, staff burnout, job dissatisfaction and low morale.

Action point 7.3 – Skill mix in my practice setting

Consider the skill mix in your practice setting. How many 'whole time equivalent' (WTE) staff are employed to work in the setting?
Overall what do you think about the skill mix in your practice setting?

The RCN (2006b) recommends a skill mix ratio of 65 per cent RNs to 35 per cent CSWs as a benchmark for general hospital wards. In other practice settings, however, such as intensive care areas, a much higher ratio is necessary. WTE relates to the total number of staff hours expressed as a percentage of full-time positions. For example a nurse who works full-time (37.5 hours per week) would be expressed as 1.0 WTE. A nurse who works 30 hours per week would be expressed as 0.8 WTE and so on.

Recruitment and retention of staff

Identifying appropriate numbers of qualified and unqualified staff required to deliver a service is only one part of the equation in the management of human resources as team members can be mobile in that they may apply for promotion, retire or leave because they are not getting job satisfaction in their current duties. The DCM needs therefore to be knowledgeable with regard to the retention and recruitment of staff.

Various reports have indicated that healthcare staff are highly dissatisfied with aspects of their work, and that improvements need to be made to retain staff (e.g. Meadows et al., 2000; Finlayson et al., 2002). A staff survey is also conducted and published each year by the Healthcare Commission (2007). Key findings for mental health and learning disability trusts for instance, in 2006–07, are as follows:

- 68 per cent of staff regularly work more than their contracted hours in a week, including 54 per cent who regularly work unpaid extra hours – both slight decreases on previous years.
- 9 per cent of staff had experienced some sort of discrimination at work, compared with 8 per cent in 2005.
- 73 per cent of staff indicated that they were generally more satisfied than dissatisfied with their jobs, the same as in 2005.
- 22 per cent of staff had experienced physical violence from patients or their relatives, and 1 per cent from other staff – these figures were unchanged from 2005.
- 34 per cent of staff had experienced bullying, harassment or abuse from patients or their relatives (a slight increase since 2005), and 16 per cent from other staff (compared with 15 per cent in 2005).
- 31 per cent of staff had witnessed at least one potentially harmful error, near miss or incident in the 12 months before the survey, although this figure has decreased substantially over the past four years.

Recruitment and retention of staff is also highlighted by the *Wanless Report* (HM Treasury, 2002), as noted in Chapter 1, which emphasised the need for concerted longer-term planning for the NHS workforce.

Action point 7.4 – Promoting staff retention

What is the rate of staff turnover within your practice setting or your organisation? This relates to the number of staff who leave the organisation each year, expressed as a percentage of the overall workforce. What initiatives are you aware of that have been implemented to promote staff retention? You may find it helpful to look at the IWL (DH, 2000b) publication.

Relevant areas of IWL with regard to family friendly employment are discussed in the next chapter.

Organisations and their employees – expectations of each other

To be able to function effectively as teams and individuals, organisations and individual members of staff have certain expectations of each other. In addition to contractual commitments, the employee also has other expectations of the organisation, such as the provision of a safe working environment. The employing organisation also has certain expectations of their employees.

 Action point 7.5 – Employer-employee expectations

Consider this notion of expectations and compliance within your own organisation, and make notes on what you as an employee expect from the organisation that employs you, and what the organisation expects from you?

There are likely to be a range of expectations by both parties in the employee-employer relationship. This is referred to as a *'psychological contract'* that involves a process of giving and receiving by the individual and by the organisation. It covers a range of expectations, rights, privileges, duties and obligations, which have a significant influence on people's behaviour but which are not in the form of a written agreement.

You may have included some of the following within your list of employee expectations:

- Provide safe and hygienic working conditions
- Make every reasonable effort to provide job security
- Attempt to provide challenging and satisfying jobs and reduce alienating aspects of work
- Adopt equitable personnel policies and procedures
- Allow staff genuine participation in decisions that affects them
- Provide reasonable opportunities for personal development and career progression

- Treat members of staff with respect
- Demonstrate an understanding and considerate attitude towards personal problems of staff.

The nature and extent of individuals' expectations vary widely, as do the abilities and willingness of the organisation to meet them. Expectations also change over time, and they are part of the social responsibility of management and are in addition to any statutory requirements placed upon the organisation. IWL standards (DH, 2000b) identify some of the employee expectations that employers should endeavour to meet.

The organisation on the other hand expects the employee to adhere to a number of rules and regulations that will be agreed and signed as part of the employment contract. Furthermore, the employer expects the employee to fully accept the established philosophy of the organisation, and contribute to the achievement of its objectives; to be loyal to the organisation when on and off duty; and not to abuse facilities that the employee is entrusted with.

In the context of the organisation's expectations and requirements from their employees, Stewart (1993) also focuses on employees' loyalty to organisational goals. She identifies a number of ways in which an organisation can achieve this (also referred to as theory Z), which are:

- long-term employment;
- a unique philosophy and clear statement of objectives;
- intensive socialisation of recruits;
- staff mobility through job rotation, and therefore more generalist rather than specialist skill, resulting in slower promotion;
- an appraisal system that emphasises individual performance and longer-term goals to gauge where the employee wishes to be some years hence;
- emphasis on work groups, but being non-directive once a task has been assigned;
- open communication encouraging contacts with other departments;
- consultative decision making; and
- showing concern for the employee by managers spending substantial amount of their time talking to employees about what matters to them.

Managing non-human resources effectively – budgets and budgeting

A range of non-human resources are available to the DCM to deliver care and treatment in their practice settings. This section therefore provides an overview of how 'money' is spent on healthcare, and to do so explores budgeting by looking at what a budget is, why prepare budgets, the different approaches to budgeting, and the likely advantages and disadvantages of each approach in healthcare organisations. The DCM has to be aware of the costs of care and treatment and the need to ensure financial viability and to achieve targets. The DCM's role in budget management is to ensure they are managing within existing resources. So what are the sources of financial resources for healthcare?

Sources of NHS income and expenditure

Money for the annual NHS budget is generally drawn from:

- Tax revenues – approximately 85 per cent
- National Insurance contributions – approximately 9 per cent
- Other sources such as charges to patients, for example, prescription charges.

Resources are allocated as 'revenue' and 'capital' funding. *Revenue funding* is money that is used for day-to-day running costs of the area of practice such as expenditures on salaries, and consumables such as medical and surgical supplies, heating, lighting and drugs. *Capital funding* is the money that is allocated for the purchase of:

- items which have a life of more than one year; and
- items of equipment which cost, either individually or as a group of related items, more than £5000.

Any item of plant or equipment that meets either or both of these conditions may be called a capital item, tangible asset or fixed asset, and capital funding includes earmarked or ring-fenced funding.

Thus, more than 90 per cent of NHS income comes from DH, and is allocated to trusts via SHAs. The rest is either donated by outside organisations or generated by the healthcare trust itself, and includes gifts and bequests (trust funds), and loan income (to self-governing trusts only).

Generated income – Money that is raised by healthcare organisations, from the level of NHS Trusts to individual wards or departments. It includes:

- Private patients' fees
- Rents from land and premises
- Income from retail sites on hospital premises that pay a fee to the unit for using of their facilities
- Money received from the sale of buildings, land and/or capital items
- Money raised from diverse things such as lease of space on the ward for advertising, hiring of a room.

Gifts and bequests – These can be donations of money or equipment to a specific unit, individual or organisation. It includes legacies, gifts and appeal funds sometimes for pre-identified specific purposes, for example, research, or continuing education for staff in the area. A problem with this is that sometimes they are donated as capital items but without the revenue funding to support their use.

Loans – Directly Managed Units are not entitled to receive loans as they must operate on the above sources of income. However, trusts can borrow money if a monthly shortfall is predicted especially when approaching the end of the budget year. Self-governing trusts may arrange to obtain loans, but have to pay interest on them.

NHS funding is gradually changing to 'payment by results' (DH, 2007f). This new way of funding comprises hospitals and other providers being paid for the clinical activities undertaken rather than 'block agreements'. They are commissioned by PCTs for the volume of activity required to deliver services, and is based on standard national price tariff, but adjusted for regional variations in wages, for instance.

Budgeting – what is it and why explore it?

DCMs have to be aware that there is a set budget for delivering care in their practice setting. So what is a budget and what does the DCM need to know about budgeting? A budget can be defined as a set amount of money identified in advance of a period of time for spending on a particular set of activities that reflect the agreed policies and strategies necessary to meet the objectives of the organisation.

One of the reasons for exploring budgeting is that managing human and non-human resources is an essential managerial role for DCM's as identified in Chapter 2, and by Mintzberg's (1990) as a 'resource allocator'. It involves deciding where, what and how resources will be deployed, and what other resources are needed.

Other reasons for preparing organisational budgets are to:

- determine income and expenditure as precisely as possible with the available information;
- identify organisational objectives and priorities, noting some expectations may not be met;
- communicate plans and coordinate activities;
- authorise expenditure and activity; and
- measure performance against objectives.

Budgeting also needs to be examined in the context of government policy, accountability and monitoring.

i   *Policy* – A budget explains to the person responsible for controlling expenditure, not only how much money has been allocated over a specific period of time, but also for what purposes that money has been allocated, that is, the resources it is intended to purchase. The budget also indicates the relative importance given to different clinical services (in terms of the amount of money to be spent on them), and is therefore a statement of policy.

ii *Accountability* – Once a budget has been created, responsibility for managing the money and resources is delegated. There is usually a hierarchy of responsibility, but each person in that hierarchy becomes accountable for the money and resources allocated.

iii *Monitoring* – A budget breaks down expenditure month by month, and by monitoring the amount of money that is being spent, it is possible to assess each month whether a practice setting has spent more or less money than it has been allocated.

Budgeting at ward/local level

A monthly statement of expenditures is usually despatched to designated clinical managers identifying the exact amount of money spent on their ward or unit. So what are the items you would expect to see listed in the statement? Box 7.1 identifies the key items in a monthly budget statement for a practice setting indicating items or activities on which money was spent in the preceding month.

Box 7.1: Key items in the monthly budget

Pay expenses	Non-pay expenses
• Nursing staff on various pay bands, and manpower equivalent hours worked • Agency staff used • Clerical staff wages • CSWs on pay bands 2 or 3	• Drugs • Dressings • Medical consumables • Equipment and medical devices

---

The monthly budget also shows the total amount spent during the month, and therefore also the amount overspent or underspent.

Budgeting is also used in long-term planning, to work out the financial effects of, for example, the purchase and running of a large piece of equipment in a practice setting, or the provision of a new service. Some flexibility needs to be built into the budget in case expenditure in one area requires cutbacks in another.

Approaches to budgeting

There are three principal approaches to devising budgets for each financial year. These are (i) activity-based budgeting (ii) incremental budgeting, and (iii) zero-based budgeting, which are briefly explored forthwith.

Activity-based budgeting is the approach that the DCM is most likely to have some involvement in. It entails estimating the volume and nature of the planned workload, identifying the fixed costs necessary to operate the planned workload, calculating the detailed and total costs of each 'unit' of work and setting the budget by multiplying the planned activity by the unit cost.

Applied to the practice setting, activity-based budgeting thus can involve estimating for instance how many episodes of different operations will be carried out by the Day Surgery Unit, or how many immunisations need to be performed at a particular health centre, during the forthcoming financial year, and the cost of the resources that will be required to perform them effectively.

The advantages of activity-based budgeting are that:

- the budget is set with a clear view of the workload expected;
- it has some flexibility built in to reflect actual workload;
- actual unit costs can be compared with planned unit costs (standard costs) to monitor the efficiency of the service; and
- it enables management to focus on efficiency (unit costs) and on controlling fixed costs within the budget rather than on workload over which they may have less control.

The disadvantages of activity-based budgeting include the following:

- identifying simple measures of workload is difficult, as the actual cost of each unit is rarely standard;
- unit/standard costs based on historic costs may not provide a measure of efficiency;

- variable cost elements of budgets must be recovered by additional contract income, or else there will be an overspend;
- fixed costs are often fixed only in the short term; and
- relatively sophisticated information systems are required.

Incremental budgeting involves ascertaining the actual necessary budget for the current financial year, and increasing it by a percentage approximating the prevailing inflation rate, but without non-recurring costs. Anticipated new activity or agreed changes in service need to be allowed for, and an inflation reserve in case it rises during the financial year.

Recurring items include all activities of the current financial year. Non-recurring items at trust level include for instance if the Accident and Emergency department is being closed down at one healthcare trust because it is being moved to another.

Inflation reserve includes pay awards and price indices. Approved variations to budgets include additional contract income due to increased workload and items released from reserves. They can also be:

- changes to services agreed during the year;
- recognition of unfunded workload pressures; and
- extraordinary circumstances, for example, costs due to fire or flood damage.

There are advantages and disadvantages in each type of budgeting. The advantages of incremental budgeting are that they are:

- easy to operate and understand;
- undemanding on management and time; and
- can operate even with weak information systems.

The disadvantages include:

- changes in activity/mode of delivery are not always reflected in the budget;
- it can perpetuate inefficient use of resources; and
- there is a lack of ownership of budgets by managers responsible.

Zero-based budgeting involves costing every item of resource, human and non-human, ascertaining the need for each of them in the forthcoming year, and costing them anew every time. This means identifying the quantity and quality of various services required, and then building up a budget from a zero base with optimum staff numbers and paybands, consumables, equipment and accommodation.

Zero-based budgeting is used for instance, when a new outpatient's clinic is being planned for a particular healthcare site. The advantages of zero-based budgets are that they:

- are directly linked to the quality of service required and the planned level of activity;
- encourage efficiency and discourage incremental budgeting;
- are usually realistic and achievable; and
- managers take ownership of them.

The disadvantages are that they can be very time consuming and expensive to constitute, there is a danger of 'reinventing the wheel', and there can be a lack of certainty about budgets year on year.

Budgeting considerations

In addition to the approaches to budgeting just detailed, there are other important considerations regarding budgeting that are now examined.

a) *Planning*: There are two main elements of planning:

1 strategic planning which refers to planning that identifies a long-term view of the objectives for services in the locality – this can be for five, ten or fifteen years; and

2 operational planning which refers to planning on a day-to-day, month by month basis.

b) *Considering effectiveness and efficiency*: These terms were defined earlier in this chapter, and are at the very heart of accountability of the budget-holder for justifying how allocated money is spent.

c) *Prioritising*: Healthcare practitioners need to be aware that budgeting usually takes into account the activities that are highest priority, and they are allocated monies in preference to those classed as lower priority.

d) *Budget statements*: Budget holders and budget managers generally receive a monthly statement from the finance department indicating usually in retrospect the amount spent on various items during the preceding month. It highlights areas of overspend as well as underspend (see Box 7.1).

e) *Matching supply and demand for CPD*: A certain amount of money is always allocated for the CPD of qualified and unqualified healthcare practitioners. Healthcare organisation's training budgets may be held centrally with individual practice settings meeting the costs of staff replacement for members who are away on study leave. The budget needs to be spent appropriately in ensuring that they meet the costs of the course that equips or updates employees in areas of skill or knowledge that are vital for meeting patient care needs.

f) *Problem-solving and decision-making*: Managers are normally equipped with skills and resources for attending to unanticipated eventualities that surface during day-to-day healthcare activities. They have to be resolved as they occur bearing all possible consequences in mind.

g) Providing leadership by practising what one preaches.

Managing non-human resources – equipment, consumables and clinical guidelines

Of the seven groups of resources required for achieving the healthcare organisation's goals, buildings, equipment, information technology, consumables, human resources, methods (i.e. procedures, protocols and guidelines) and money (BEICHMM), human and money resources have been discussed in detail so far in this chapter. The relevant key items were identified in Box 7.1 in the monthly budget statement. The remaining resources in this acronym are now examined.

Buildings, equipments and consumables

There are a number of reasons for the buildings of healthcare organisation to be adjusted, be they hospitals or smaller units, with time. Often driven by government policy to deliver a more patient-centred and more efficient service, new departments and units may be built, and others closed. They, however, need to meet various legal requirements, such as health and safety and energy efficiency.

Equipment such as those for performing electrocardiographs, electro-convulsive therapy, relaxation therapy, hoists for moving and handling, beds or cots and so on are purchased to aid patients' recovery. They have to be regularly checked for safety as guided by various health and safety acts and regulations, such as *Provision and Use of Work Equipment Regulations* (HSE, 1998). Medical devices such as glucometers, intravenous fluid administration devices, and their attachments also have to be purchased and stocks replenished. Consumables also include single-use items such as dressings, stationery, medications, intravenous administration sets and disposable gloves and aprons.

Procedures, protocols and clinical guidelines

To ensure the clinical activities of the healthcare organisation are performed to the highest standards, trusts need to have well-established clinical protocols, clinical guidelines and procedures as resources that support healthcare delivery. Each of them need to be reviewed by a pre-determined date, but are usually continually updated with addenda based on new evidence for changes.

The benefits of having protocols and clinical guidelines, and the potential problems with them, were discussed in the context of ensuring quality of healthcare in Chapter 5. Procedures need to be performed in the context of an individualised, holistic and evidence-based approach to care.

Guidelines for efficient and effective resource management

The characteristics of an effective organisation are dependent upon the effectiveness of all its managers, including the DCM fulfilling his or her managerial roles (as detailed in Chapter 2) effectively. Guidelines for effective and efficient use of resources in healthcare are as follows:

- Review budget statements each month to monitor expenditure.
- Where you identify areas of overspend, discuss possible ways to reduce the overspend with your manager and ask them if you can shadow them when they meet with the finance manager.
- When a vacancy arises, review the post to ensure that the replacement post meets service requirements rather than replacing like with like automatically.
- Establish the unit cost of consumable resources and raise awareness amongst the team.
- In instances of acute staff sickness, look at working within existing resources in the first instance rather than automatically requesting temporary staffing.

- Discuss productivity with your manager and team members to consider how it could be improved (see *The Productive Ward* in Chapter 5).

Chapter summary

This chapter has examined the resources required for effective healthcare delivery, which entailed examining:

- the human and non-human resources that are required by the healthcare organisation to achieve its goals; the question why 'manage' resources was addressed after identifying present day actual healthcare expenditure; how resources are managed;
- managing human resources, which incorporate skill mix, staff morale as well as recruitment and retention of staff;
- managing non-human resources, which included an examination of budgets and budgeting, the sources of NHS income, the reasons for exploring budgeting, different approaches to budgeting and budgeting at ward/local level; and
- managing other non-human resources such as equipment, medical devices and consumables, as well as clinical guidelines, protocols and procedures; guidelines for efficient and effective resource management were also presented.

EIGHT Strategies for personal and peer support

Introduction

Over the years, healthcare professions have been identified as some of the most stressful occupations (e.g. Meadows et al., 2000; Leners et al., 2006; RCN, 2006b), and healthcare practitioners therefore need to develop effective and positive coping strategies to enable them to fulfil their duties without avoidable anxiety, and with support mechanisms to manage challenging situations. This chapter examines the availability of organisational, personal and peer support mechanisms for healthcare practitioners, and how they can be utilised for not only preventing or dealing with such situations, but more importantly to perceive them as learning opportunities. This chapter addresses this aspect of the management role, and incorporates peer-learning and peer-review, which provide healthcare practitioners with a medium for gaining external impressions of their level of knowledge and competence, and possibility for identifying further learning needs. They provide healthy means for obtaining feedback, and also bring with them several benefits as well as fulfil other recommended professional requirements.

Chapter objectives

On completion of this chapter you will be able to:

- indicate why support mechanisms are important components for healthcare practitioners to deal with the challenges that they encounter in their day-to-day clinical activities;
- analyse formal support mechanisms in healthcare such as the role of the Occupational Health Department, clinical supervision and peer support networks; and
- identify informal peer support mechanisms in healthcare, their significance, recommended techniques for implementing them and their strengths and weaknesses.

Why support mechanisms for healthcare practitioners

There are several reasons for examining the personal and professional support mechanisms that are available to healthcare practitioners. This section addresses those reasons.

Challenges in the healthcare professions

Duty clinical managers, like the majority of healthcare professionals, have continuing demands made upon them by a number of stakeholders, both during a span of duty, and over longer periods of time. This is in addition to their clinical intervention functions towards patients in their care. Specific examples of such demands are identified in Figure 8.1.

You should be able to add to diagram 8.1 elements that are specific to your practice setting and specialism. At times unexpected violent episodes by patients or relatives in the Accident and Emergency Department for instance, or an unexpected death in the practice setting could prove emotionally demanding, and mechanisms for a debrief following such incidents can prove beneficial. Various sources of stress can be identified, such as:

- Worklife imbalance
- Working with temporary staff (e.g. agency nurses)
- Lack of availability of resources
- Competing demands for time
- Paperwork and bureaucracy
- Staffing challenges such as sickness and vacancies
- Professional relationships
- Lack of team work
- Cliques
- Capacity issues
- Inefficient systems of work

Figure 8.1 *Demands on DCMs*

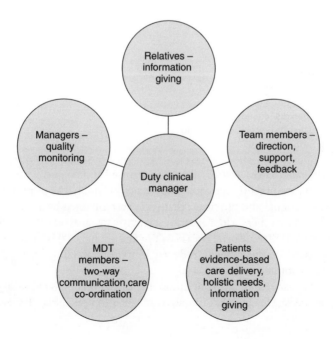

- Clinical incidents
- Shift work
- Off-duty
- Changes
- Redeployment
- Lack of job security
- Lack of job availability
- Financial constraints
- Restructuring.

For community nurses, sources of stress can include heavy clinical caseloads, and the knock-on effects of general practitioners being under pressure to meet government health targets. There's a feeling that workload has increased, and peer contact diminished as workload has shifted from secondary to primary care, and has become more high-tech community care. Evans (2002) explored district nurses' experiences of stress at work, and found that the most stressful aspects of work for this group of district nurses were: work overload, climate of change, nursing patients with complex care needs, lack of team work with other departments, and their family–work interface. Previously, Ballard (1994) reporting on a RCN-supported study found considerably higher levels of work-related stress and sickness absence amongst district nurses than for nurses in general, and even higher than in the general working population. Poor managerial support and lack of availability of counselling were causes of further dissatisfaction.

Hawkins and Shohet (2006) suggest that stress is a state of fatigue, ill-health and at times depression caused by distressing, strenuous and emotionally overwhelming situations. They identify various symptoms of stress (p. 27), including:

- Overtiredness
- Loss of appetite
- Insomnia
- Headaches or migraine
- Diarrhoea, indigestion
- Inability to concentrate
- Paranoid thoughts
- Avoiding friends/ colleagues
- Increased alcohol intake, overeating
- Sudden mood swings.

However, if experiences of stress are not recognised and no positive action is taken, then the healthcare practitioner could experience burnout. The term burnout refers to a state of emotional and physical exhaustion accompanied by a lack of interest in one's job, low trust in others, a loss of caring, cynicism towards others, self-deprecation, low morale and a deep sense of failure (Hawkins and Shohet, 2006). Such consequences could be avoided or their effects reduced if appropriate support mechanisms or structures are instituted and functional.

Another likely source of stress or emotional demand is bullying or aggression in the workplace. A survey by NHS Employers (2006a) revealed high levels of bullying in NHS trusts. NHS Employers (2006b) indicate that bullying in the NHS may be characterised as offensive, intimidating, malicious or insulting behaviour, an abuse or misuse of power through means intended to undermine, humiliate, denigrate or injure the recipient. Practical steps that can be taken to combat bullying include those suggested by Randle et al. (2007) as:

- disclosing to a friend or trusted colleague;
- exploring knowledge of workplace policy, and discuss with a trade union representative;
- maintaining a written log or diary of bullying incidents; and
- being assertive and recognise your's and others' rights.

Specific guidelines on bullying at work are available from the RCN (2005c), UNISON and other trade unions. Excessive levels of such demands are difficult to meet within paid working hours and various concerns may pre-occupy the manager long after they have gone off-duty from the practice setting. Over prolonged periods of time, these may lead to the healthcare practitioner experiencing stress and even burnout.

 Action point 8.1 – My own sources of support

Make a list of who you turn to for support when uncertain about (a) a professional issue, (b) a personal issue.

The support structures available to you are likely to include work colleagues, family members and friends. These support mechanisms can be grouped under formal and informal mechanisms. These are discussed shortly.

There are several ways in which healthcare practitioners can develop positive coping mechanisms to prevent or deal with stress. These include exercise, eating healthily and looking after your personal own health, as opposed to negative strategies such as smoking and drinking excessively. Instead of complaining among friends and being a victim, healthcare practitioners can take proactive actions, and explore potential ways of resolving challenging situations such as by working differently, utilising team meetings, reflecting on practice, supporting team members and recognising stress in them. Sickness management and treating staff fairly and equitably are approaches that DCMs can adopt towards their juniors.

Staff satisfaction at work

As noted in chapter seven in its annual staff survey, the Healthcare Commission (2006) identified several problematic aspects of working in healthcare organisations. Without adequate support, such problematic encounters can be causes of stress and burnout.

One of the mechanisms that is used periodically (usually annually) by organisations to gauge staff morale and how far job expectations are being met is through staff satisfaction surveys. The organisation can thereby gain feedback from their workforce on various aspects of working life. The surveys can include open and closed questions on the following aspects.

- Existence, clarity and strategies for achieving the organisation's vision
- Extent of top-down, bottom-up and peer communication
- Learning and development opportunities
- Availability of IDPRs
- Opportunities to use own initiatives
- Career opportunities
- Health, safety and welfare in the working environment
- Stress and availability of counselling
- The general physical environment of the workplace
- Harassment and bullying
- Staff involvement in decisions
- Feedback on performance
- Diversity and equality
- Management of change.

Thus, staff satisfaction surveys can include questions on harassment and bullying at work, and if they do exist, then there can be questions on whether they were reported, and what the outcomes of reporting were. If they are not reported, then the reasons for this can be explored. Staff dissatisfaction at work can be the cause of experiences of stress.

 Action point 8.2 – Staff satisfaction surveys

Explore when a staff satisfaction survey was conducted at your place of work, which office it was initiated by, whether it was anonymous, and what the outcomes were. Alternatively, access the Healthcare Commission website and view the most recent staff survey for your organisation to ascertain its content.

Staff satisfaction surveys comprise a useful means of gaining employees' perspectives on aspects of the workplace and inherent dynamics that they are happy with and those that are more problematic.

On countenancing the above-mentioned challenges, healthcare practitioners may wish to explore their thoughts with peers or seniors with appropriate knowledge. Such a milieu or vehicle can be available through formal support mechanisms and more informal ones; some are well-instituted organisationally, and others are potentials in that they are at developmental stages.

Formal support mechanisms

The formal support mechanisms available for health professionals can be at individual, organisational and supra-organisational levels. Such support can be gained from:

- line managers;
- working spans of duty that accommodate family commitments;
- the Occupational Health Department;
- clinical supervision;
- reflection-on-action mechanisms;
- professional forums;
- peer-learning;
- mentorship; and
- buddy systems.

Line managers

Line managers' roles include staff support in that the DCM should provide appropriate support to those who they manage, and also expect support from their own line managers.

Accommodating other commitments

One of the most significant staff support strategies identified in *The NHS Plan* (DH, 2000a) is that the NHS will invest in its staff in ways that enable them to lead balanced working lives. How this can be achieved is documented in *Improving Working Lives Standard* (IWL) (DH, 2000b) which is a blueprint by which NHS employers and staff can measure the management of human resources. Organisations are given Kitemark® certification against their ability to demonstrate a commitment to improving the working lives of their employees.

IWL is based on the premise that improving the working lives of staff contributes directly to better patient care through improved recruitment and retention; and also patients have stated that they want to be treated by well-motivated, fairly rewarded staff (DH, 2000b). It indicates that the way NHS employers treat staff will later be part of their core performance measures and linked to the financial resources they receive. Consequently, NHS employers were instructed to create well-managed, flexible working environments that support staff, promote their welfare and development, and respect their need to manage a healthy and productive balance between their work and their life outside work. According to IWL, this can be achieved by:

- HR Strategy and commitment to support service targets;
- team-based employee self-rostering;
- annual hours arrangements;
- childcare support;
- reduced hours options;
- flexi-time;
- carers support;
- career breaks;
- flexible retirement;
- building a diverse workforce that reflects the local community;
- changing the long hours culture;
- healthy workplace commitment;

- managers leading by example;
- finding out what working arrangements work for staff;
- challenging traditional working patterns;
- involving staff in the design and development of better, flexible working practices;
- conducting annual staff attitude surveys – asking relevant questions and acting on the key messages;
- HR policies and processes that make a difference to individuals;
- reducing staff turnover; and
- accessible training and development packages for all staff.

NHS employers are expected to provide for all these components which include high profile activities such as childcare support and flexible working hours. IWL standards were to be achieved by NHS employers providing evidence of commitment to improving the working lives of their staff in the following components:

- recognising that modern health services require modern employment services by having a HR strategy in place for the organisation to deliver against *The NHS Plan* targets, *National Priorities and Working Together* targets;
- understanding that staff work best for patients when they can strike a healthy balance between work and other aspects of their life outside work by demonstrating leadership from the top and Board commitment to more flexible, supportive, family friendly and culturally sensitive ways of working and training;
- accepting a joint responsibility with staff to develop a range of working arrangements that balance the needs of patients and services with the needs of staff, by finding out what working patterns staff can/prefer to work;
- Values and supports staff according to the contribution they make to patient care and meeting the needs of the service by staff across the organisation from all disciplines and irrespective of their role in the organisation or working patterns, demonstrating their commitment to the organisation and feeling the organisation is committed to their well-being;
- providing personal and professional development and training opportunities that are accessible and open to all staff irrespective of their working patterns by demonstrating appropriate investment in training for staff who have patterns of working that are not standard; and
- having a range of policies and practices in place that enable staff to manage a healthy balance between work and their commitments outside work and practical support in place to meet the specific needs of staff.

Various guidelines on how different healthcare professions can achieve these components of IWL and standards have been published since the initial IWL publication.

The Occupational Health Department

Another support mechanism available to healthcare practitioners is the Occupational Health Department. The staff-support element of their remit generally includes:

- Health surveillance
- Health and safety advice
- Work station assessments

- Health education and promotion
- Counselling
- Return to work rehabilitation programmes
- Ad-hoc advice
- Sickness and absence management.

Some departments include other functions such as planning for retirement. It is through their 'counselling' and 'ad-hoc advice' that occupational health services provide individual personal support to healthcare practitioners. Individuals can be referred to a staff counsellor if more specialist support is required. They can provide advice for work-related issues via telephone or on a 'drop-in' basis.

Clinical supervision

One of the most widely advocated particular forms of organised individual and peer support is clinical supervision. This section explores what clinical supervision is, the aims and benefits of clinical supervision, how clinical supervision can be implemented and the likely problems that need to be addressed beforehand.

The NHS Management Executive (1993) indicated that clinical supervision is a formal process of professional support and learning which enables individual practitioners to develop knowledge and competence, assume responsibility for their own practice and enhance consumer protection and safety of care in complex situations. Nicklin (1995) for instance defined clinical supervision as a facilitated process during which the nurse reflects on their practice, analyses issues and problems, clarifies goals, identifies strategies for goal-attainment and establishes an appropriate plan of action.

Essentially, clinical supervision allows a registrant to receive formal professional support in the workplace by an appropriately skilled clinical supervisor. Regular pre-arranged meetings are held which enable the supervisee to identify areas of professional development for both self-improvement and enhancement of patient care. According to the NMC (2006a), clinical supervision enables registrants to:

- identify solutions to problems;
- increase understanding of professional issues;
- improve standards of patient care;
- further develop their skills and knowledge; and
- enhance their understanding of their own practice.

The NMC (2006a) recommends that:

- every registrant should have access to clinical supervision and each supervisor should supervise a realistic number of practitioners;
- preparation for supervisors should be flexible and sensitive to local circumstances;
- the principles and relevance of clinical supervision should be included in pre-registration and post-registration education programmes; and
- evaluation of clinical supervision is needed to assess how it influences care and practice standards; evaluation systems should be determined locally.

Similar arrangements can apply to allied health professionals. The NMC also indicates that clinical supervision should be available to registrants throughout their careers so they can constantly evaluate and advance their professional knowledge and skills. Along with the PREP (continuing professional development) standard, the NMC (2006b) also sees clinical supervision as an important part of the clinical governance agenda.

The NMC supports the principle of clinical supervision but believes that it is best developed at a local level, and therefore does not advocate any particular model of clinical supervision, nor provides detailed guidance about its nature and scope. Instead, the NMC has defined a set of principles that could underpin any system of clinical supervision, which are:

- Clinical supervision supports practice, enabling registrants to maintain and improve standards of care.
- It is a practice-focused professional relationship, involving a practitioner reflecting on practice guided by a skilled supervisor.
- Registrants and managers should develop the process of clinical supervision according to local circumstances. Ground rules should be agreed so that the supervisor and the registrant approach clinical supervision openly, confidently and are aware of what is involved.

However, Shanley and Stevenson (2006:586) suggest that clinical supervision is a 'multi-meaninged phenomenon defined through the context of its use'. It is important to note that supervision is a concept that prevails in various arenas, within and outside healthcare. Midwives for instance, have a system of statutory supervision through Local Supervising Authorities, as detailed in the *Midwives Rules and Standards* (NMC, 2004b). It is used beneficially in varied fields such as social work, counselling, education, probation, police and even for refugees and asylums seekers, that is, in most 'people professions' (Hawkins and Shohet, 2006:ix).

The anticipated benefits of clinical supervision are that it should lead to improved job satisfaction through greater empowerment, and improvement in the quality of patient care. However Driscoll (2000) suggests that the term clinical supervision does not explicitly signify what its advocates define it as. The term clinical supervision itself may be misleading and perhaps 'clinical support' or 'peer-supervision' might be more appropriate. Another possible weakness of clinical supervision is that some healthcare practitioners are apprehensive about it, fearing that it could be associated with some type of inspection of individuals' weaknesses as a management-led function that is designed to control rather than facilitate.

Furthermore, some healthcare practitioners fear that managers could link clinical supervision with IDPR, although this notion is firmly discarded by the advocates of clinical supervision in nursing (e.g. Darley, 1995, a then professional officer at the UKCC). This is because it may be perceived by employees that if objectives set in IDPRs are not achieved for whatever reason, then the reviewee may be deemed incompetent, and this can lead to disciplinary procedures being invoked. The intention of clinical supervision is to use supportive, clinically legitimate and confidential ways of aiding healthcare practitioners identify professional development needs and means of achieving them. It is thus a constructive medium for assisting individuals with practice deficits to improve their practice voluntarily. Other barriers to clinical supervision include:

- pressure on time that can be used on direct patient care;
- too few adequately trained supervisors;
- cost in terms of time allocated;
- exercise of 'position power' if the supervisor is of a more senior status; and
- availability and accessibility of supervision.

If the supervisor–supervisee relationship breaks down, this can be problematic as well. Furthermore, with regard to confidentiality as governed by the NMC (2008a) *The Code – Standards of Conduct, Performance and Ethics for Nurses and Midwives*, nothing that happens during supervision should be revealed to others without the explicit consent of the supervisee. If a record of supervision is maintained, it should be the property of the supervisee, and likely to be retained in their own portfolio. However, as in other situations, if during supervision a practitioner discloses a breach of the code, then confidentiality cannot be assured.

Clinical supervision can be conducted at individual or one-to-one level with a more experienced healthcare practitioner supervising a junior. Alternatively, it can constitute peer-supervision, which is peer-led, group or team supervision. This should be non-competitive, clear and with well-focused objectives.

Group supervision, however, can vary to some extent from one group to another. Sloan and Watson (2002) note that in group supervision the clinical supervisor facilitates a group of four to six supervisees. Facilitation and helping skills are prerequisites which can be acquired through appropriate training, even in pre-registration nursing courses as reported by Carver et al. (2006).

The facilitation of clinical supervision needs to be systematic through the use of a model of clinical supervision. Two popular models of clinical supervision are Proctor's (2001) three-function interactive approach and Heron's (1989) six-category intervention analysis framework.

Use of these models need to be supported by the conditions for a therapeutic relationship, which include acceptance, genuineness and empathy (Rogers and Freiberg, 1994). These are essential components of 'helping' (a term often used interchangeably with counselling), and counsellors and psychotherapists value supervision from peers. However counselling is a deeper and much more complex process than supervision, and therefore supervision sessions must not be interpreted as counselling.

Proctor's (2001) model entails three main functions of clinical supervision, namely normative, formative and restorative.

A normative function	Addresses the quality control aspects of practice as well as managerial aspect related to policies and procedures, developing standards and clinical audit.
A formative function	Refers to the educational process of skill development, including EBP.
A restorative function	Providing supportive help for those working with regard to stressful situations, with the aim of enabling the professional to understand and manage these situations during professional practice.

This model constitutes a framework that enables both parties to focus on the purpose of the activity. Sloan and Watson (2002) argue that Proctor's model is not too prescriptive, and therefore allows leeway, but at the same time gives insufficient guidance to supervisors, especially in the restorative component. Heron's (1989) six-category intervention analysis model provides another suitable framework, as identified in Chapter 1.

Various studies, such as those by Wheatley (1999) and Bowles and Young (1999), have highlighted the benefits of clinical supervision. Hyrkas et al. (2005) found that clinical supervision has long-term positive effects on an individuals clinical practice and self-development. However, in a review of clinical supervision in nursing, Jones (2006) and Bishop (1998) amongst others highlighted issues with clinical supervision. Jones (2006) for instance notes that the implementation and utilisation of clinical supervision is haphazard, and the processes are little understood.

However, Leners et al. (2006) extend the concept clinical supervision further, and suggest that in view of sporadic inadequate staffing, and negative knock-on effect this has on desired patient outcomes and on nurses' job satisfaction, a career-long mentorship programme should be established for nurses at various stages of their professional careers. The term mentorship thus extends the concept beyond how it is currently utilised through episodic clinical supervision, to interactions and relationship between mentor and mentee on a more continuous basis, and thus 'empower, inspire, guide, advise and model clinical behaviours that promote quality patient care outcomes in a team-based work environment' (p. 653). Clinical supervision often involves reflective learning which is discussed in Chapter 11.

Non-formal and informal support mechanisms

Informal modes of personal and peer support can occur through peer-review and peer-learning. It also occurs through individuals investing time and effort to impart knowledge and skills to peers and learn from each other, a notion referred to as social and human capital.

The role of peer-review and peer-learning

This section examines the role of peer-learning and similar mechanisms within healthcare professions that constitute systems of support and feedback.

The DH's (1999:30) nursing strategy document *Making a Difference* indicates that in the 'learning that takes place at work through experience, critical incidents, audit and reflection, supported by mentorship, and clinical supervision and peer-review can be a rich source of learning'. Thus when the healthcare practitioner is allocated a new activity or project, they might feel that they will benefit from sounding their thoughts out informally with trusted and appropriately knowledgeable colleagues or peers. Peer-review can be utilised for benchmarking purposes, or for exchange of protocols and clinical guidelines between peers at different healthcare trusts. A peer may be:

- a colleague of equal status in the same practice setting;
- a colleague of equal status from another practice setting in the same specialism or department;

- someone of higher status in the same practice setting or another practice setting in the same specialism;
- someone of equal or higher status from another hospital; or
- an individual in a very similar or identical vocation, and perhaps also from a similar social background and age group.

Davies (1990) suggests that peer-learning fosters activities to help creativity. For instance, access to the Internet in the practice setting for literature searching and locating critically reviewed material can itself constitute informal peer-education – available in the practice setting's resource room or the staff room for informal social learning, or in the post-graduate department. Goldsmith et al. (2006) report on a formal peer-learning strategy through partnering first year and third year student nurses for clinical practice sessions. Both groups of students indicated this as 'a positive learning experience'. Yuen Loke and Chow (2007) also report on positive effects from similar arrangements. Campbell et al. (1999) report on a study that discusses the successful implementation of peer-education approaches to behaviour change in health education. Peer-learning is also discussed in the context of social and human capital shortly in this chapter.

For student nurses, practice educators can arrange regular 'student support meeting' in healthcare organisations, whereupon all practice setting are notified, and since students have supernumerary status, they can usually be released to attend.

Related to peer-learning is the concept of synergogy, as suggested by Mouton and Blake (1984). Synergogy comprises a deliberate plan designed to enable very small groups of learners who have good rapport with each other and are on the same programme of learning, to learn from each other, and not to have to learn from an educator if they see the latter as an authority figure. This concept is also based on an interpretation of synergy which suggests that significant learning takes place when two or more individuals study together than when they do so separately. The learning is supported by learning materials being managed by a learning administrator.

 Action point 8.3 – Synergogy and protected time for learning

The notion of protected or allocated time specifically for CPD is gathering momentum. With libraries and other learning facilities, including electronic databases, increasingly being instituted in healthcare organisations, can you envisage if and how synergogy can be organised by groups of healthcare practitioners of equal status, and used efficiently?

Peer-learning can be based on self-assessment. The development of professional knowledge and competence by individuals as lifelong learners is usually based on self-assessment (Gopee, 2000), but self-assessment in isolation is not sufficient for learning and development, and individuals at times look to their peers for their views and judgements. Hollis (1991:47) asserts that while 'self-monitoring is a useful tool, it can be unrealistic and does not overcome the problem of learners needing the intellectual stimulus of others and acquiring subtle insights from peers'.

Jarvis and Gibson (1997) observe that during one's career, as healthcare practitioners become more skilled and autonomous, the less likely/frequently they are to be assessed by others. For several practice nurses for instance, Cairns (1998:24) indicates that because they work autonomously or in isolation, they need the mechanism of clinical supervision for peer-feedback. The same may apply to clinical nurse specialists whose roles also provide marked autonomy. The DH (1999) identifies professional autonomy as both a privilege and a significant responsibility that has to be matched by commitment to public accountability.

Considering the likely strengths and weaknesses associated with peer-assessment, one of the strengths is that it constitutes an opportunity to the healthcare practitioner to practice a skill in a safe environment, and to receive instant feedback on performance (this feedback has impact). The likely weaknesses include the probability of individuals being overcritical, their own lack of knowledge of the skill area, the possibility of disagreement between peers and even the lack of or unavailability of peers or of opportunities for peer-assessment.

On the other hand, Jarvis and Gibson (1997) draw attention to other risks of peer-assessment such as being a case of the 'blind leading the blind', and therefore unsafe practice may continue. However, Welsh (2006) argues that peer-assessment comprises an essential transferable skill. Peer-assessment is part of professional regulation or self-regulation which is a requirement for all healthcare professions (e.g. GMC, 2006).

Peer-review on the other hand, lies at the foundation of professional accountability and autonomous practice in healthcare delivery. It is an inherent component of clinical governance, clinical supervision and several other quality related activities. It can be initiated and implemented at one-to-one, departmental or organisational level.

Malby and Manning (1998:24) report on an inter-trust peer-review learning network whose key principles include participants being keen to 'learn and support others in an atmosphere of trust and openness'. A collaborative, non-competitive learning environment at all levels of the organisations is also seen as important. They conclude that peer-review 'can make a valuable contribution to organisational and personal development and professional practice' (p. 25).

As to what to review, some other activities that may benefit from peer-review include:

- determining evidence of professional updating – in clinical activities, managerial, and clinically or work-based teaching;
- post-conference reflections;
- exploring accountability towards various parties, such as the profession, the public, the employer; and
- self-assessed further developmental requirements.

Malkin (1994) reports on several advantages of peer-review, including:

- improvement in standards of care;
- increased awareness of personal professional accountability in practice;
- identification of personal areas of strengths and weaknesses; and
- stimulating professional development and decentralisation of power throughout the organisation.

The GMC (2007) has advocated peer-review in various areas of medicine, including in relation to performance assessment of doctors when concerns have been expressed in relation to their competence.

Empirical evidence of the effectiveness of peer-review is variable. McAllister and Osborne's (1997:40) study indicates that peer-review 'increases personal accountability and has demonstrated improved quality of care and clinician performance'. The following constitute guidelines for good practice for peer-review.

- Ascertain assessment or performance criteria prior to the event.
- Be skilled in feedback giving, as well as using trigger phrases for giving feedback identified by Bond and Holland (1998).
- Always be sensitive to the assessee's or reviewee's responses, verbal and non-verbal, to the feedback being given. The degree to which weaknesses are pointed out straight after the performance must be balanced to prevent being overcritical.
- Be objective as the assessee may feel he/she is already fully aware of weaknesses of the performance being assessed.
- Additional written constructive feedback can also be given, for a complete picture.
- Always encourage self-assessment prior to peer or assessor feedback.
- Strict use of Rogers and Frieberg's (1994) acceptance and warmth, empathy and genuineness, is important.
- Need to be a skilled facilitator to ensure damage is not being done to the assessee if the peer-assessment is being formally assessed.
- The facilitator role is to guide and support peers, and enable them to develop self-confidence.
- Consider recording the peer-review centrally so that action plans, improvement and progress can be recorded. This can be private or open to inspection (Pedler et al. 2001).

Peer-review is increasingly becoming a part of autonomous practice and professionalism. Garbett et al. (2007) report on a study of peer-review facilitated by the 360-degree feedback method (discussed in Chapter 3), suggesting that this facilitates collection of evidence for clinical expertise development, and also might contribute to improved working relationships. However, being a relatively novel idea in most nursing circles, initial participation in peer-review should be introduced as a highly recommended but voluntary and consensual activity.

Professional forums

Another vehicle for peer-reviews are professional forums, which comprise special interest groups that are convened based on clinical specialisms. The RCN, for example has approximately 85 of these forums, which can provide a supportive medium for peer-consultation.

Social and human capital as peer-learning mechanisms

Another increasingly recognised means of peer support and peer-learning involves the notion social and human capital, which comprises the ad-hoc or informal support that individuals give to and receive from course peers, friends, colleagues and even families. Social capital refers to time, patience, sharing information and teaching that individuals 'invest' in each other in relatively closely knit social groups and amongst peers. The influence of clinical colleagues, co-students and personal relations on learning is thus as significant and valuable. Putnam (1993) suggests that social capital is characterised by:

- the existence of community networks;
- local identity and a sense of solidarity and equality with other community members; and
- norms of trust and reciprocal help and support.

Field (1999:12) asserts that a great deal of learning is social in nature, and connected to this is the gap in current knowledge as to the level of informal learning that occurs as and when people: '... learn in corridors, over tea, in the car park, as well as through unnoticed patterns of behaviour and interaction in the classroom itself', although the amount and effects of this mode of learning is difficult to quantify. Practitioners on the same course, for instance, meet socially or e-mail each other to share articles and references related to module assignments, thus forming informal networks that facilitate learning.

Social and human capital therefore entails the social investment of personal time and knowledge, that can enable the continuation of professional learning, which is a feature that clinical managers can support and further develop to enhance learning. Moreover, social capital thrives in settings that constitute learning organisations, which are inherent features of lifelong learning. The work environment in which the healthcare practitioner delivers care seems to have considerable effect on their learning, as discussed in Chapter 11. Bahn (2001:115) discusses this in the context of social learning theory, and notes that the social environment has considerable impact a on 'collaborative approach to learning through the use of peers and expert practitioners as role models'. Even crisis situations comprise fertile grounds for novel ideas and methods to develop. It seems that Coleman's and Baron et al's suggestions should be endorsed and the notion cultivated. Such conditions seem to be germinating already within networks of friends or colleagues, and need to be recognised.

Thus, infrastructures and facilitatory mechanisms often unbeknown to employers seem to support lifelong learning for the registrant, and the practice setting ultimately benefits from them. Social capital is also related to the concept of the 'informal organisation' which Mullins (2007) and others identify as non-formal structures that constitute a powerful force in shaping cultures in organisations.

Colleagues may encourage learning and development with an enquiring mind by bringing back appropriate literature acquired from conferences and workshops. These can be made available in the practice setting as learning materials. Colleagues who have been on CPD courses and who subsequently share aspects of what they have learnt perhaps by giving a talk or facilitating a workshop to disseminate their knowledge.

A seemingly equally important factor, is the role played by non-healthcare individuals such as parents, friends and the individuals' partners or spouses in the context of the external perspectives that they might provide, and can constitute instigators or supportive mechanisms for learning. Social and human capital is also reflected in doctors influencing healthcare practitioners' learning as they work on joint projects such as setting up specialist clinics or on an RCT.

Consequently, Watkins and Marsick (1992:115) suggest a redefinition of human resource development with 'greater inclusion of informal and incidental learning strategies' by personnel responsible for this role. Peers and managers could therefore appreciate the contribution of social and human capital to learning, that is, of the 'informal' modes, and accommodate mechanisms to facilitate this whenever they can, as ultimately patient care is enhanced through better informed care. Baron et al. (2000:38) explored the concept from various standpoints in the general literature, and suggest that in the spirit of the 'current questing age', the concept should neither be dismissed as an empty vessel, nor overblown as a concept that will address all social issues.

Guidelines for effective peer support

- Encourage formal and informal peer-learning.
- Implement and sustain clinical supervision either on a one-to-one basis or as group supervision.
- Use and encourage use of the healthcare organisation's support mechanisms.
- Normalise reflection-on-action.
- Ensure annual IDPRs are conducted.
- Ensure colleagues know of other management support anchors other than the line manager.
- Always maintain confidentiality.
- Encourage colleagues to be members of professional special interest groups.

Chapter summary

This chapter has explored the key components of personal and peer-support strategies available to healthcare practitioners. This included the following:

- the reasons for support mechanisms being important components of healthcare organisations, including enabling healthcare practitioners to deal with the challenges that they encounter in their day-to-day clinical activities with positive coping mechanisms; and staff satisfaction at work;
- formal support mechanisms which include the role of Occupational Health Departments, clinical supervision and reflective practice, and the availability and accessibility of support mechanisms; and
- non-formal and informal support mechanisms, including the role of peer-learning, peer-assessment and peer-review, the distinction between these mechanisms, the likely strengths and weaknesses with them, and recommended techniques for implementing them; professional forums and the concept of social and human capital. Together with guidelines for effective staff support.

It is clear from the discussions so far in this chapter that one of the benefits of peer-support mechanisms are that they constitute a medium for proactive and informal learning, and for healthcare practitioners to develop personal management plans to avert or manage stress.

NINE Patient involvement, participation and partnership

Introduction

Patient-focused services and patient choice are central concepts to the government's modernisation of health and social services. The achievement of this vision is dependant upon a change in culture, together with a shift in power base to empower patients to become more actively involved both in the development of services and in the care that they personally receive. The DCM needs to keep abreast of policy developments; evaluating the implications for their practice setting and identifying ways of applying relevant ideologies to their everyday clinical practice. This chapter begins by contextualising the motivating forces for the development of choice and consumerism, together with the promotion of more patient-focused health and social care services.

Chapter objectives

On completion of this chapter you will be able to:

- identify the policy and professional drivers for the development of patient-focused services, choice and the promotion of consumerism within healthcare;
- examine the power base that underpins the practitioner–patient relationship;
- define person-centred care and identify prerequisites and barriers to the application of this concept to clinical practice;
- explore the concepts of patient involvement, participation and partnership and their application within the context of your professional practice; and
- reflect on current practice and identify strategies to enhance person-centred care within your clinical area.

Background to patient involvement, participation and partnership

Political and professional drivers, coupled with increasing public expectation, have created a demand for the provision of more patient focused services. The advent of the initial *Patient's Charter* (DH, 1991) promoted the concepts of individualised, patient-centred care and heralded the beginning of the government's commitment to provide patients with rights regarding the healthcare services that they receive. Patient choice has more recently emerged as a central theme and it is anticipated that it will act as a catalyst for improving both the quality of service provision and patient outcomes. The Government advocates that 'patient involvement improves patient satisfaction and is rewarding for professionals' (DH, 2004d:1). Wanless (HM Treasury, 2002) suggests that providing patients' with choices and facilitating them to be more actively engaged in their healthcare is potentially a more cost-effective strategy compared to more passive patient roles.

The NHS Plan (DH, 2000a) introduced a vision for the modernisation of the NHS with an underlying shift in power from healthcare practitioners to patients. The *NHS Improvement Plan* (DH, 2004b) set out priorities for the NHS to enable it to become a 'personal health service for every patient'. The White Paper *Choosing Health* (DH, 2004e) set out the government's strategy for supporting people to make healthier decisions, through better information, advice and personal support; it further placed onus on the responsibility of the individual for personal health.

More recently the *Your Health, Your Care, Your Say* (DH, 2006f) consultation identified that the public want to have more personal control over their healthcare together with care provided closer to home. The resultant white paper outlined three themes as being central to the government's vision for the strategic direction for health and social care services in the community, namely 'putting people more in control of their own health and care', 'enabling and supporting health, independence and well-being' and 'rapid and convenient access to high-quality, cost effective care' (DH, 2006b:13). The government's choice agenda, however, can conversely be seen as a way of introducing market forces within the health economy. This promotion of consumerism, where patients can choose between service providers for elective surgery, to include a choice of public providers together with a private provider, will drive competition between healthcare providers with resultant anticipated improvements in quality. In addition to elective surgery, the choice agenda has also been applied to long-term conditions through the *Expert Patient Programme* (DH, 2001a).

High Quality Care for All (DH, 2008a) was published alongside a draft constitution for the NHS (DH, 2008b); the draft constitution sets out further rights and pledges for patients based around the following areas:

- access to health services,
- quality of care and environment,
- nationally approved treatment, drugs and programmes,
- respect, consent and confidentiality,
- informed choice,
- involvement in healthcare and the NHS, and
- complaint and redress.

The constitution also sets out responsibilities for patients and the public with the intention of supporting the NHS to work effectively together with responsible resource utilisation.

Such policy initiatives support the move from traditional paternalistic approaches of healthcare to a more empowering approach that encompasses both individual responsibility and choice. Other examples of available choice options include whether to give birth at home, in a birthing centre or in hospital, and also opportunities to self-refer to therapy services, such as physiotherapy. A NHS website is available to provide patients with information about health and choices that are available to them.

NHS Choices can be accessed at http://www.nhs.uk/Pages/homepage.aspx and includes, amongst other features, the opportunity to compare hospitals by the treatment they provide and the facilities that they offer.

The DCM needs to be politically aware and to evaluate the impact of national and local policy on care delivery within their practice setting and has a responsibility to ensure that individualised patient-centred care, underpinned by choice, is central to the care that is provided.

Patient and public involvement

The government advocates that patient and public involvement should be part of everyday practice in the NHS (DH, 2005b), and has identified a number of principles that underpin the delivery of patient-led services. These are outlined in Box 9.1.

Existing mechanisms to support patient and public involvement within the NHS are highlighted in Figure 9.1 and are summarised below:

- Patient Advice and Liaison Service (PALS) – NHS Trusts are required to provide a PALS service for patients and their carers, to act as a point of contact for information, advice and advocacy. PALS can also support problem resolution, signpost patients to sources of independent advice and advocacy, and provide a source of feedback to the healthcare trust.
- Local Involvement Networks need to be provided in each area that is served by a local authority with responsibility for social services. Their roles are set out in

---

Box 9.1: Principles underpinning the delivery of a patient-led service

1 Respect people for their knowledge and understanding of their own experience, their own clinical condition, their experience of the illness and how it impacts on their life.
2 Provide people with the information and choices that allow them to feel in control.
3 Ensure everyone receives not just high quality clinical care but care with consideration for their needs at all times.
4 Treat people as human beings and as individuals, not just people to be processed.
5 Ensure people always feel valued by the health service and are treated with respect, dignity and compassion.
6 Understand that the best judge of their experience is the individual.
7 Ensure that the way clinical care is booked, communicated and delivered is as trouble free as possible for the patient and minimises the disruption to their life.
8 Explain what happened if things go wrong and why, and agree the way forward.

(Adapted from DH, 2005b)

Figure 9.1 *Mechanisms to support patient and public involvement*

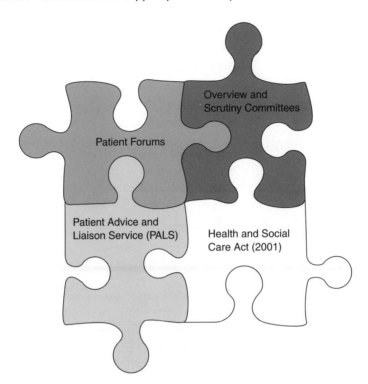

legislation, their primary function being to enable individuals and groups to influence the planning, commissioning and delivery of local care services.

- Health and Social Care Act (DH 2001a) – Section 11 of this Act places a duty on the NHS to consult patients and the public in the planning and development of health services, together with proposals affecting the way that services operate.
- Overview and Scrutiny Committees – local authority councillors have the powers to review and scrutinise the planning, provision and operation of the health service and to make recommendations for improvement.

We have thus far explored the national agenda with regard to the modernisation of health services to support the government's vision for a patient-led NHS. We will now relate this concept to the role of the DCM within everyday clinical practice.

Involvement, participation and partnership

The concepts involvement, participation and partnership are relatively broad, and therefore are open to interpretation and are often used interchangeably (Roberts, 2002). Cahill (1996:563) asserts that 'there is no clear consensus on what patient-participation entails' and goes on to say that as a result of this lack of clarity the concept has become '... rhetoric or even a cliché'. Cahill (1996) argues that a hierarchical relationship exists between the three concepts of involvement, participation and partnership (Figure 9.2). Within this hierarchy Cahill states that, patient

Figure 9.2 *A hierarchical relationship between concepts (adapted from Cahill, 1996)*

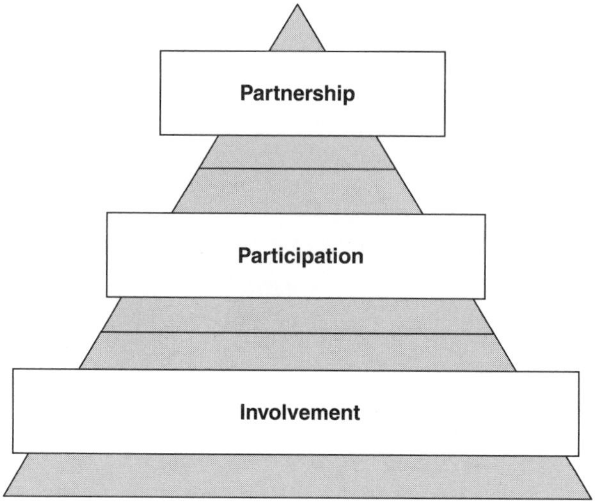

Partnership

Participation

Involvement

involvement or collaboration is a prerequisite for patient participation, which in turn is a prerequisite for patient partnership.

The first concept, patient involvement, is comparatively more passive in nature where, for example, the healthcare practitioner may provide information or elicit information from the patient as part of the assessment process. Participation, on the other hand, necessitates more active involvement from the patient; an example of which is where the healthcare practitioner engages the patient in an evaluation of his or her care. Working in partnership, however, is premised more upon equality within the patient–healthcare practitioner relationship, an example of which is 'contracting' with a patient through goal setting, or the development of a care, therapy or birth plan.

The degree to which equality can be achieved within the healthcare practitioner–patient relationship, however, has been questioned. Within the hierarchy of concepts, Cahill (1996), for example, considers partnership as more idealistic and not necessarily achievable in practice and concedes that there is a need, therefore, to establish the extent to which patients want to participate in their care. Conversely, Tutton (2005) identified participation as a process that occurs in the context of care giving, rather than within a hierarchy of decision-making.

 Action point 9.1 – Applying patient involvement, participation and partnership to the DCM role

- Draw a table with three columns, at the top of the columns insert one of the concepts of involvement, participation, partnership, one in each column.
- For each concept record a list of examples of how you apply this, or could apply this, within your role as DCM.

Within the concept analysis of patient participation completed by Cahill (1996), she identified a number of defining attributes, without which, she argues, the concept might not have surfaced. These attributes are:

1 the presence of a relationship between healthcare practitioner and patient;
2 a narrowing of relevant information, knowledge and/or competence gap between healthcare practitioner and patient;
3 a surrendering of a degree of power or control by the healthcare practitioner;
4 engagement in selective intellectual and/or physical activities during some of the phases of the healthcare process; and
5 a positive benefit is associated with the intellectual and/or physical activity.

Of the five defining attributes that Cahill (1996) identified, the presence of a relationship between healthcare practitioner and patient emerged as the most important. Within the patient–healthcare practitioner relationship, however, it needs to be acknowledged that some patients are supportive of healthcare practitioners making decisions on their behalf and respect the professionalism of the healthcare practitioner to act in their best interests.

Roberts' (2002) study, for example, identified that 60 per cent (18 of 30) of patient participants stated a preference to be involved in decision-making, with 23 per cent (7) stating that they did not want to be, predominantly on the grounds of their ill health. The healthcare practitioner must acknowledge the uniqueness of each patient and recognise the necessity to treat patients as individuals, establishing the degree to which they want to participate in decisions about their healthcare.

Action point 9.2 – Power and the healthcare practitioner–patient relationship

- Consider who is more powerful, the patient or the healthcare practitioner.
- Make a list of sources of power for each of these two groups.

Boxes 9.2 and 9.3 provide examples of potential sources of power for healthcare practitioners and patients, respectively. When sources of power are evaluated, the DCM needs to identify ways of shifting the balance of power more in favour of the patient.

Box 9.2: Potential sources of power: healthcare practitioners

Sources of power	Healthcare practitioner
1 Knowledge and expertise	• Professional education • Clinical experience

---

Box 9.2: Continued

2	Language	•	Medical terminology
3	Environment	•	Delivering care/therapy/treatment within the environment of a healthcare institution
4	Uniform	•	Represents status
5	Professional autonomy	•	Gatekeeper to treatment/care/therapy

---

Box 9.3: Potential sources of power: patients

Sources of power		Patient
1 Knowledge and expertise	•	Information technology e.g. internet
	•	Impact of their illness on their everyday experiences
2 Environment	•	Care/therapy/treatment delivered within the patient's own home
3 Rights	•	Choice of care provider
	•	Right to complain
	•	Right to ask for a second opinion
	•	Right to refuse treatment

Power can form a significant role in the healthcare practitioner–patient relationship. Transfer of power from healthcare practitioner to patient, however, is not without challenge as it is at odds with more traditional, paternalistic approaches to care delivery where healthcare practitioners act/acted in the best interests of patients. Within contemporary practice, altering the power base more in favour of the patient will necessitate a change in culture. It needs to be recognised that power can be exerted both consciously and subconsciously, and that some healthcare practitioners will adapt more readily than others.

Decision-making needs to encompass choice; with the healthcare practitioner outlining the various options that are available to the patient. EBHC, however, can sometimes be dichotomous with 'patient choice'. A NICE guideline, for example, may indicate a particular type of treatment or therapy; conversely, the patient may express an alternative preference. Part of the initial patient assessment needs to be the identification of the individual patient's wishes regarding their preferred level of participation in their healthcare.

Brashers et al. (1999) indicate that research shows the existence of a dichotomy between the amount of healthcare information that patients consistently report that they would like, and the number of questions that they actually ask during consultations. It must, therefore, also be recognised that preferred level of participation may be affected by a number of variables and may change at different points within the patient journey.

Person-centred care

The terms 'patient-centred care', 'personalised care' and 'individualised care' consistently feature within government documents regarding the modernisation of both health and social care services. Within the *Essence of Care* (DH, 2003), the term 'person-centred' is used to signify 'activities that are based on what is important to a person from their own perspective'. Within the *National Service Framework for Older People* (DH, 2001b) person-centred care has been defined as treating people as individuals and providing them with choices regarding their care. This definition includes two key words, namely 'individual' and 'choice'. Figure 9.3 illustrates the HEART Choice Model that has been developed from concepts identified within the literature, which includes a number of key concepts that are central to the healthcare practitioner–patient relationship in supporting the achievement of person-centred care.

Each of the concepts within the HEART Choice model will now be explored individually:

Holism:	Encompasses regard for the 'whole person', both physically and psychologically. Within a holistic approach, physical, social, psychological, spiritual and cultural issues are recognised as having collective impact on the well-being of the individual.
Empowerment:	To empower is to provide power or authority to another person. This term is both widely and liberally used in everyday practice,

Figure 9.3 *Concepts that support person-centred care*

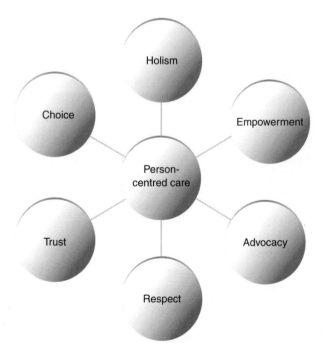

however, often with lack of regard as to the conceptual complexities involved in truly empowering patients.

Advocacy: An advocate is someone who acts on behalf of another person. The advocate needs to understand the values, beliefs and perspectives of the person whom they are representing. Conflicting roles and responsibilities of healthcare practitioners need to be acknowledged, for example, those relating to their role of professional carer versus their role as an employee of the healthcare organisation. It must also be acknowledged that, within the healthcare practitioner–patient relationship, the level of advocacy required will vary from patient to patient and will be dependent upon a number of factors such as the preference of the individual patient.

Respect: To respect is to have positive regard for another person. Mutual respect and positive regard should ideally be evident on both sides of the healthcare practitioner–patient relationship.

Trust: Trust relates to the reliability of another person and having confidence in them. Within the healthcare practitioner–patient relationship, the patient must be assured that the healthcare practitioner will address their best interests.

Choice: Is having the opportunity to select a preference from a range of alternatives. At a more 'micro' level within the healthcare practitioner–patient relationship, the healthcare practitioner must strive to identify everyday choices that they can provide their patients with in relation to their care/therapy.

The HEART Choice model can be used to inform the achievement of true patient-centred care within everyday practice and can be applied at all levels within the organisation.

 Action point 9.3 – Patient-centred care from rhetoric to reality

- Consider each of the six concepts that make up the HEART Choice model.
- For each concept, compile a list of examples of how you apply the concept within your interactions with patients.
- Within your role as DCM, as discussed in Chapter 2 for instance, you have a responsibility to monitor and supervise the care delivered by members of your team. Make a list of strategies that you can employ to facilitate the delivery of person-centred care within your practice setting.

Strategies for promoting person-centred care

Everyday clinical practice presents a wealth of opportunities for healthcare practitioners to promote person-centred working. Central to this approach, however, is the need to complete a holistic assessment that clearly identifies the values, beliefs and concerns that are important to the individual patient. Assessment skills are fundamental to the professional practice of all healthcare practitioners. Patient assessment presents a unique opportunity to provide the foundation for person-centred working. It could be argued that a skilled assessor can engage in a 'conversation with a purpose' with his/her patients to elicit personalised information, as opposed to asking them a list of predetermined questions in the order in which they appear within the assessment document. The opportunity for self-assessment can also be considered where the patient can be supported to complete their own assessment, recorded in their own words. Once a holistic assessment has been completed, the healthcare practitioner should strive to engage the patient in the planning, delivery and ongoing evaluation of their care.

Action point 9.4 – Person-centred assessment

- Reflect on a patient assessment that you have completed recently. How confident are you that within the assessment you identified what the patient considered to be important to them, such as their values, needs, problems, concerns and goals?
- Make a list of the strategies that you used to elicit the patient perspective, such as open questions, managing the environment to promote privacy and open body language.
- Think of ways that you could further enhance your practice in the achievement of person-centred assessment.

Practice examples that support person-centred working are outlined below; further opportunities such as case conferences, ward rounds, goal setting, ICPs and multi-disciplinary team meetings will be explored in Chapter 10.

A ticket to go home

She's Got a Ticket to … Go Home (IHI, 2006) is an initiative that originates from America where patients are provided with an individual whiteboard in their room that details information regarding what they need to achieve prior to being discharged home. This provides a practical tool that acts as a mechanism for three-way communication and engagement between the patient, their family/carer and healthcare practitioners. Within the United Kingdom, the essence of this approach is transferable; however, to maintain confidentiality, a person-held record may be more appropriate than an individual white board.

Patient diary

The use of a patient diary presents the healthcare practitioner with an opportunity to learn from the everyday experiences of the individual patient, and to use this information in meeting their personal care/therapy needs. This approach is sometimes used within palliative care where the patient uses a diary to record symptoms, emotions and problems, for instance. The diary can be used to identify problems and needs and the impact on the individual, to monitor care and to solve problems.

The 'Single Assessment Process'

The 'Single Assessment Process' (SAP) was introduced through the *National Service Framework for Older People* (DH, 2001b), the purpose of which is to ensure that older people receive appropriate, effective and timely responses to their health and social care needs, and that professional resources are used effectively. SAP aims to:

- provide person-centred assessment and care;
- ensure older people receive appropriate, effective and timely responses to their health and social care needs;
- prevent practitioners duplicating each other's assessments and the care they provide;
- prevent people having to repeat the same information again and again;
- ensure that information is shared (with the individual's consent) between agencies and departments;
- create a person-held record of information about the individual's needs and the care and service they receive; this will reduce the amount of time practitioners spend finding and collating information and ensure any decisions are based on all of the information available; and
- ensure all agencies have shared values and approaches to assessment, care planning and care provision so that people will receive a similar assessment experience wherever they are assessed.

SAP is an evolving process and has been acknowledged as best practice for the assessment of adults regardless of age. Work is currently going on to look at the development of a Common Assessment Framework across the DH and other government departments; and the process associated with SAP is central to this work. This will also encompass the care programme approach that is used within mental health, together with the person-centred approach that is used within learning disability.

Achieving person-centred care – patients with special needs

Within healthcare there are a number of patients who may need more specialist consideration and support in identifying and meeting their personal values, beliefs and needs. Patients may include those who, for example, are unconscious or those who experience a cognitive impairment or other mental health problem, communication deficit or learning disability. Kitwood (1997), for example, states that for people who experience advancing cognitive impairment, the aim of person-centred care is to 'maintain personhood'. Kitwood states that personhood implies 'recognition, respect and trust' and defines personhood as '... a standing or status that is bestowed upon one human being by others in the context of relationships and social being'. Strategies to support the achievement of person-centred care in more specialist circumstances can include biographical approaches and advance directives.

Biographical approaches

Biographical approaches can support the achievement of a person-centred assessment for patients, who for example, may have a cognitive impairment or learning disability. Within this approach, individual patients are afforded the opportunity to share their life experiences to provide insight into their values, needs and aspirations. A small-scale study completed by Clarke et al. (2003) identified that the use of a biographical approach can promote person-centred care through enhancing the personhood of the older person. Clarke et al. (2003), however, recognise the resource limitations of adopting this approach in everyday clinical practice and suggest that rather than being an activity in its own right, the approach can be integrated into everyday care activities, such as, supporting the patient with their activities of daily living.

Advance directives

An advance directive, also known as a living will, enables a competent individual to out-line the treatment and care that they would like to receive in the future, should they subsequently lose the capacity to decide or to communicate their preferences. The Mental Capacity Act (HMSO, 2005) provides a statutory framework that aims to protect vulner-able people who may be unable to make decisions on their own behalf. The Mental Capacity Act (HMSO, 2005) includes statutory rules that govern advance decisions to refuse treatment and outlines 'formalities' that need to be complied with, which include that the decision must be in writing and signed and witnessed and that a statement must be included that states that the advance decision stands 'even if life is at risk'.

Challenges to the achievement of person-centred care

The achievement of person-centred care can pose challenges for the healthcare practitioner, some of which are directly related to individual practice, others that are affected by the prevailing culture of the clinical environment within which they work, and others that relate to resource constraints. Challenges to the individual can include their personal values, attitudes and beliefs and the influence that these may have on their care/therapy delivery, such as in a situation where the healthcare practitioner is a non-smoker and the patient who is pregnant, or has continuous obstructive pulmo-nary disease, chooses to continue smoking.

Challenges relating to the culture of the clinical environment can include routine working practices, such as an expectation by the day staff that the night staff will complete a number of bed-baths before shift handover. Challenges relating to the availability of resources can include environmental factors, such as having a limited number of side rooms or showers, or relate to consumable resources such as the type of toiletries and hospital clothing available to the patient, or to care-rationing decisions that have to be made due to pressure on resources, for example, the amount of therapy time that a patient receives or whether a nurse washes a patient rather than promoting their independence and supporting them to wash themselves.

 Action point 9.5 – Personal, cultural and resource challenges to person-centred care

Draw a table with three columns, and label the columns 'personal challenges', 'cultural challenges' and 'resource challenges'. Consider the challenges that you

Action point 9.5 – Continued

face as a healthcare practitioner in the provision of person-centred care to your patients and record these within the first column. In the second column make a list of challenges to the achievement of person-centred care that emanate from the culture of the practice setting where you work. In the third column record the challenges that are posed through limited availability of resources. Next to each of the challenges that you have identified, record two or three potential solutions. Solutions can be based on you as an individual working differently or may require the support of your manager and colleagues in changing the working practices within your practice setting. Now consider your role as DCM and the extent to which you can have a positive impact in promoting person-centred care during the spans of duty where you are 'in charge'.

Webster (2004) identified a number of factors as having a negative impact on an individual's sense of self and their personhood, namely:

- Stereotyping
- Labelling
- Depersonalisation
- Stigmatisation
- Ageist attitudes and beliefs
- Changes in health status
- Lack of 'real' choice and autonomy
- Physical environment
- Rigid organisational boundaries/service access criteria
- Task orientation based on routine and tradition
- Lack of knowledge, skills and insight by care givers.

Action point 9.6 – Balancing safety and patient preferences case study

Brenda is a 79-year-old widowed lady who was admitted to hospital after sustaining a fractured neck of femur. Brenda has a history of recurrent falls and has recently been diagnosed as having dementia. Following surgery to have her hip fracture pinned, Brenda experienced some initial medical problems from which she is now recovering. She has started to take a few steps with her walking frame and the supervision of one member of staff. Prior to admission, Brenda lived alone in a ground-floor council flat – her home for the past 30 years. Brenda has expressed a wish to return to her flat, once she is discharged. Members of the inter-disciplinary team, however, are concerned about Brenda's preferred discharge destination and have reservations regarding her safety and ability to cope at home. Key concerns centre on Brenda's short-term memory problems and her risk of falls.

1 What factors need to be addressed as part of the decision-making relating to Brenda's pending transfer of care?

Action point 9.6 – Continued

2 What strategies could you use to promote Brenda's safety while also meeting her personal wishes regarding her preferred discharge destination?
3 What support could you draw upon from colleagues, other agencies and services?

You may have identified some of the following within your answers:

- the need to establish whether or not, at this point in time, Brenda has the capacity to make the decision about discharge destination;
- if it is deemed that Brenda lacks capacity to make this decision at this point in time; that any subsequent actions taken are in her best interests, and that family members are consulted if this is the case; it would also need to be established whether there is someone who holds a lasting power of attorney that would allow them to act on Brenda's behalf if appropriate; or if Brenda has no family or friends to support her, a decision may need to be made regarding whether the appointment of an Independent Mental Capacity Advocate is required to represent her;
- use of advanced technology, such as community and social alarms (e.g. Telecare), that utilise communications and sensing technologies such as fall, flood and gas detectors;
- provision of an intensive care package that may include night sits;
- sheltered housing options; and
- allocation of a care-coordinator.

Healthcare practitioners face numerous dilemmas during the course of their everyday professional practice. They can sometimes demonstrate paternalism in the decisions that they make, which may be due to the need to maintain safety and to reduce risks, although there is a need to balance risks against the preferences of the individual. Similarly patient preferences and choices made may be at odds with evidence-based approaches to healthcare, such as if four-layer bandaging may be the evidence-based treatment indicated to promote the healing of a leg ulcer; the patient, however, may refuse this treatment and request an alternative course of treatment. Similarly, a pregnant woman may request an elective caesarean section where there is no evidence to support this approach and natural delivery would be considered appropriate. Acknowledging, respecting and treating the patient as a person are fundamental to a patient-centred model of care delivery. It is important that the implications of various treatment options are explored and that the individual is aware of any actual and potential risks associated with the various choice options that are available. In some instances, the option preferred by the patient may not be available to them either because it is not evidence-based or available on the NHS.

The healthcare practitioner–patient relationship

The healthcare practitioner–patient relationship is central to healthcare practice. Interpersonal relationships between healthcare practitioners and patients humanise care and therapy through identifying with the patients' personal experiences. The nature of this relationship needs to be explored to enable the healthcare practitioners to recognise the importance of their interpersonal skills to the development of therapeutic relationships with their patients. Different types of behaviour can exert influence on the power base within the healthcare practitioner–patient relationship, namely authoritarian or democratic. Within an authoritarian approach the health-care practitioner assumes a more powerful position and informs the patient of interventions, treatments and the outcomes of decisions made regarding their care. Within a democratic approach, the healthcare practitioner adopts a more patient-centred philosophy; identifying individual preferences and promoting choice and empowerment.

Priorities can differ between the healthcare practitioner and the patient. A patient presenting with respiratory insufficiency due to myasthenia gravis, for example, may identify social responsibilities such as providing for his family and caring for his wife and new-born baby as his main concern in the advent of an impending deterioration in condition. Healthcare practitioners may be more likely however to prioritise the need to maintain oxygen perfusion. This case scenario illustrates the need to identify the patient perspective to elicit values, goals and priorities to inform the provision of personalised care.

Within the literature there exists a plethora of studies that illustrate how the patient perspective can commonly contrast to that of the healthcare practitioner. A study conducted by Florin et al. (2005) found that nurses were less likely than patients to identify problems relating to nutrition, sleep, pain and emotions/spirituality. The study also identified that in relation to problems that had been identified collectively with patients; nurses underestimated the severity of the problem in nearly half of all cases (47 per cent).

A study undertaken by Duxbury and Whittington (2005), similarly identified differences between staff and patient perspectives. In this instance patients identified precursors to aggressive behaviour to be environmental conditions and poor communication whereas, nurses conversely cited patients' mental illnesses as the main reason. Magnus et al. (2004) revealed that nurses' assessments compared more favourably than patients' perceptions for the majority of care interventions provided at night with, for example, 73 per cent of nurses assessing 'night rest' positively and 95 per cent for 'information and participation' positively, compared to only 51 per cent and 49 per cent respectively by patients. Healthcare practitioners therefore need to identify strategies to elicit the patient perspective throughout the patient journey.

Identifying a patient's willingness to participate

In addition to choices regarding health services, choices about health similarly need to be provided for patients. Within the public health agenda, issues of state responsi-bility versus individual responsibility, however, need to be addressed. Inequalities such as poverty and education are widely acknowledged as having a positive correlation to morbidity and mortality. Government policy is paying increasing attention to the prevention of ill health and maintenance of health. The *Expert Patient Programme*

(EPP) (DH, 2001c) promulgates self-care and self-management for patients with long-term conditions. The development of patient expertise in symptom management and lifestyle choices are key approaches within this model. The DCM can support the expert patient programme through the promotion of the role and encouraging patients to access EPP courses where appropriate. Earlier on in the chapter; treating the patient as an 'individual' and providing 'choice' were identified as central concepts to the achievement of person-centred care.

 Action point 9.7 – Patient choice

- Think about the choices that are offered to patients within your practice setting.
- Compile a list of choices and for each consider the actual extent of choice, together with any boundaries that may be present.
- Which aspects of care/therapy provision within your practice setting are governed by the needs of the individual and which are governed by the needs of the institution/practice setting?
- What further choices do you think could be offered within your practice setting?

Table 9.1 highlights the availability of choices that were identified by staff who attended a multi-disciplinary person-centred care workshop. The choices are divided into those that are governed nationally, those that are available locally within individual services, together with other preferred choices that they would like to be widely available.

Many of the choices available, however, are offered within the context of boundaries, some of which relate to resource constraints. If, for example, a patient is offered a preferred time for an intervention, this in many instances is a restricted choice as other patients may similarly opt for the same time. Healthcare staff have to try and accommodate the preferences of a number of patients simultaneously while working within available resources.

Table 9.1 *Healthcare choices*

Choices governed nationally	Local choice availability	Other preferred choices
General practitioner	Menu	Individual room
Care provider	Time of therapy	Timing of consultations
Consent or refuse treatment	Wash or shower to meet hygiene needs	Unrestricted visiting
	Patient-held records	Individual use of a TV, DVD, telephone and laptop computer

Compliance versus non-compliance

The achievement of patient compliance with treatment, therapy and advice can be challenging for healthcare practitioners. It has been identified, for example that, as many as 50 per cent of older people may not be taking their medications as intended (RPSGB, 1997). Concordance related to medicine-taking is a more contemporary approach to prescribing that involves negotiation between the patient and healthcare practitioner (Marinker et al., 1997). This approach recognises the beliefs and preferences of the patient and acknowledges that to achieve compliance, patients need to know how the medication will benefit them personally. Concordance is an example of the promotion of partnership between the patient and the healthcare practitioner.

In promoting similar approaches within other areas of healthcare practice, it is important to analyse the factors that influence individual patient decisions to comply or not to comply with treatment, therapy and advice. An ethnographical study completed by Tutton and Seers (2004) identified the powerlessness of older patients and how they continually tried to identify 'what was expected of them' and tried to 'fit in' with the norms of the ward, while simultaneously trying to get the care that they needed. Similarly, within a study conducted by Pearson et al. (2004), a patient respondent stated 'I told the nurse, I says "I don't take pain killers." I only took them in hospital to please them …'. These two studies suggest that patients comply with convention and treatment as a strategy to achieve favour or to ensure that their needs are met. Patient compliance, therefore, should not be regarded as synonymous with patient motivation.

A further challenge that healthcare practitioners can sometimes face within their professional relationship with patients is what has been termed by Stockwell (1984) as the 'unpopular patient'. Stockwell's study explored interpersonal relationships between nurses and patients in general hospital wards and identified that the 'least' popular patients identified by nurses fell into two broad categories: those who grumbled and complained or demanded attention in other ways, and those whom the nurses considered did not need to be in hospital or on a particular ward. A study conducted by Johnson and Webb (1995), similarly identified that the 'expression of evaluations of social worth' by nurses was widespread both in terms of 'good and bad patients'. Johnson and Webb, however, identified that ascribed labels could be 're-negotiated' rather than achieving permanency as implied by Stockwell.

 Action point 9.8 – Popular and unpopular patients

- Think about a patient that you have enjoyed working with.
- Make a list of the positive attributes/influences that contributed towards the positive healthcare practitioner–patient relationship in the example that you have identified.
- Now think about a patient that you have not enjoyed working with.
- Make a list of the attributes/influences that contributed towards the less positive healthcare practitioner–patient relationship in the example that you have identified.
- Now compare the two lists that you have recorded to identify any commonalities, distinguishing factors or trends.
- For the patient that you did not enjoy working with list the strategies that you employed to manage this situation.

It is important that all patients are treated as individuals and encouraged to be involved in their care and that the achievement of person-centred care transcends any issues regarding popularity or unpopularity. Chapter 8 explores a number of strategies for both personal and peer support to assist healthcare practitioners in the course of their professional roles.

Ways of coping

In addition to the challenges posed for healthcare practitioners in caring for less 'popular' patients, other groups of patients can also constitute a source of pressure. Morse et al. (1992), for example, proposed a model to describe nurses' responses to patients who are suffering. Within this model, engagement by the nurse is affected by their focus either on themselves or their patient, together with whether their response is reflexive or learned. Morse et al. (1992) identify a number of strategies that are utilised to control personal engagement with a patient who is suffering, such as pity, sympathy, consolation, compassion, commiseration and reflexive reassurance. Healthcare practitioners need to recognise the influence of their own values, attitudes and personal experiences to the quality of care that they provide.

Good practice guidelines

The following, constitute good practice guidelines for patient involvement, participation and partnership in healthcare delivery:

- Establish the patient's preferred form of address and ensure that this is documented and respected by team members.
- Ensure that patient assessments are holistic and address the individual's values, beliefs, concerns and personal preferences.
- Prepare plans of care in collaboration with patients and ensure that they are reflective of the individual's values, beliefs, concerns and personal preferences.
- Involve patients in all decisions about their care and promote informed decision-making and choice.
- Utilise biographical approaches to support the achievement of person-centred care for patients who have a cognitive impairment or learning disability.
- Talk with and listen to patients. Ask them about their experiences and evaluations of care and take positive action to address any concerns.

Chapter summary

This chapter began by contextualising the motivating forces for the development of choice and consumerism, together with the promotion of more patient-focused health and social care services. The key concepts of patient involvement, participation and partnership were then explored and applied to everyday clinical practice. The concepts person-centred care, personalised care and individualised care were analysed and opportunities identified to achieve these approaches in practice. As advocated by the Joseph Rowntree Foundation (2005) 'Involvement starts with talking but it shouldn't end there'.

The DCM needs to act as a role model to promote choice and the achievement of personalised care. To ensure that person-centred care is achieved, they need to act as a champion so that both their practice and that of fellow team members is person-centred. A wealth of opportunities exists within the practice setting to achieve this, with person-centred assessment being fundamental to success. The DCM needs to lead by example and monitor and supervise care delivery in the practice setting to ensure the achievement of patient-centred outcomes and personalised care.

This chapter has explored the key components of patient involvement, participation and partnership which impacts on the DCM's roles, and included:

- the background to patients and the public's involvement, participation and partnership in healthcare delivery;
- person-centred care including strategies to promote person-centred care, achieving person-centred care for all, including patients with special needs; and the challenges to the achievement of person-centred care; and
- the healthcare practitioner–patient relationship in the context of identifying patients' willingness to participate in safeguarding their own health and well-being, as well as compliance and non-compliance with treatment and advice given by healthcare practitioners.

TEN Uni-professional, inter-professional and inter-agency teamwork

Introduction

Maximising patient outcomes, making the best use of resources, facilitating seamless services and ensuring timely transfers of patient care are reliant upon effective team-working between primary, community, secondary and social care services.

In this chapter models of multi-disciplinary, inter-disciplinary and trans-disciplinary teamwork will be evaluated, and theories related to teamwork, such as Belbin's (1993) team roles, will be critiqued and applied to multi-disciplinary/multi-agency team-working. The reader will have the opportunity to explore both their role and that of their colleagues within the teams that they belong to and to identify mechanisms to increase their effectiveness. Strategies that capitalise upon formal opportunities for inter-disciplinary/inter-agency discussion and decision-making, such as ward rounds, goal setting meetings, multi-disciplinary team meetings and case conferences, will be appraised. Finally the chapter will progress to identify ways of evaluating team performance.

Chapter objectives

On completion of this chapter you will be able to:

- identify and analyse the nature of groups and teams, models and prerequisites for effective team-working, and identify ways in which you can maximise team performance within the teams that you belong to;
- evaluate team leadership, in the context of inter-professional/inter-agency team-working, together with the challenges to leadership and management within;
- demonstrate knowledge of the theories and practice of staff motivation and identify ways to apply them within your role in the context of uni-disciplinary and inter-professional team-working; and
- critically analyse teamwork, the role of multi-professional communication within, and reflect upon ways to evaluate the performance of the teams that you belong to.

Theories of teamwork

Teamwork is often premised to be a prerequisite for good practice within health and social care. Teams, however, can be very diverse in nature and range from uni-disciplinary teams such as those exclusively comprising of a single professional group, for example, nursing staff, physiotherapists or midwives, to inter-disciplinary teams that include representation from a range of disciplines that may transcend both health and social care, together with acute and community services.

Multi-professional teamwork is conceptualised as a key mechanism for care management within the United Kingdom. Whilst there is in existence a plethora of literature espousing the potential benefits of teamwork, empirical research in support of this is more limited. Literature regarding partnership working is emerging. However, this is based on perceptions of the values of partnership working rather than empirical evidence to support this approach. A multi-professional team approach to healthcare has developed over the last 60 years in Britain, predominantly within the fields of the care of older people (Waters and Luker, 1996) and within mental health. Although such approaches are perceived to be positive, team interaction, dynamics and a shared understanding of the roles of individual disciplines can be challenging. Each discipline has its own philosophy of care that needs to feed into the wider, shared philosophy of the inter-professional and inter-agency team.

Team-working that focuses upon the needs of the person is identified within contemporary healthcare policy as a mechanism to achieve high quality outcomes for patients. *The NHS Plan* (DH, 2000a) highlighted how traditional, hierarchical working had maintained demarcations between staff groups that had resulted in duplication of effort and the need to see a number of healthcare practitioners for some patients. Collaborative working is one of 15 leadership qualities identified by the NHS III (2006:31), the benefits of which are identified as '... delivering measurable and radical health improvements in a complex and changing health and social care environment. Effective partnership promotes the sharing of information and appropriate prioritisation of limited resources. It also supports "joined up" provision of integrated care.'

It needs to be recognised, however, that professionals can collaborate with one another without being part of a team. A healthcare professional may, for example, make a referral to a healthcare professional from another discipline who can assess the patient, provide their expert opinion and undertake therapeutic interventions. Collaboration, therefore, should be differentiated from teamwork.

Differentiating groups from teams

A group can be defined as a collective unit of people who share a common interest. A group can either be formal or informal in nature. A formal group may be configured within an organisation where there is a need to perform a specific task, for example, to develop an ICP or to develop an integrated record. An informal group will tend to develop more naturally amongst peers, for example, a group of colleagues who socialise together.

A team on the other hand takes the concept of a group further, by focusing on the interrelationship between members and is premised upon the organisation of people with a shared purpose and the way in which they work together to achieve this. Consequently, a team can be defined as a group of individuals who are conversant with the organisation's mission and aims, work together to deliver the organisation's services, and feel individually and collectively accountable for the achievement of its goals.

Within healthcare, teams have been broadly classified as project teams such as those that focus on quality improvement; and care delivery and management teams that can broadly be subdivided into three categories (Canadian Health Services Research Foundation [CHSRF], 2006), namely:

1 Patient population – for example, specialist old age multi-disciplinary team
2 Disease type – for example, stroke team
3 Care delivery settings – for example, intermediate care team.

 Action point 10.1 – A group or a team

Consider the various groups and teams that you are a member of as part of your clinical role, and for each one decide whether it is a group or a team. Think about the justifications for your decision/s and base these around the definitions that were provided earlier.

Models of teamwork

A plethora of terms are used within healthcare to denote the context within which health and social care professionals work together. Leathard (2003) has identified incongruence between definitions of teamwork and cites the example of the term 'inter' that has been used to denote working between two groups, but also to a team of individuals from different backgrounds. A number of different models for the facilitation of teamwork are also in existence. Mumma and Nelson (2002), for example, differentiate between multi-disciplinary, inter-disciplinary and trans-disciplinary models of collaborative practice. These are as follows.

1 Multi-disciplinary
- Discipline – specific goals
- Clear boundaries between disciplines
- Effective communication is essential for success

2 Inter-disciplinary
- Collaborate to identify patient goals
- Expanded problem-solving beyond discipline-specific boundaries/work

3 Trans-disciplinary
- Blurring of the boundaries between disciplines
- Flexibility to minimise duplication of effort

 Action point 10.2 – Team map

Figure 10.1 provides diagrammatic representation of a multi-disciplinary team with a central focus on the patient. Consider the various members that make up your clinical team, and draw a diagram to illustrate this. Where does the patient sit within the team? Now consider the interrelationship between team members, and make notes on which of the models of collaborative teamwork outlined by Mumma and Nelson best reflects your team. Consider your team in the context of its interrelationship with other teams, both within your organisation and with external organisations.

Figure 10.1 *Members of the multi-professional team*

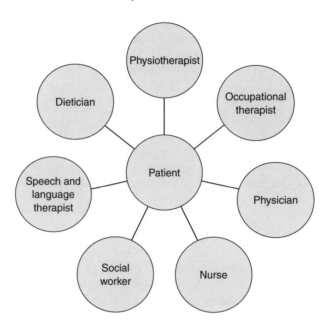

The team map that you have plotted will be beneficial for you to refer back to throughout the remainder of the chapter.

Benefits of teamwork

A number of positive outcomes have been identified from working in a team that include job satisfaction, turnover, effectiveness, innovation and patient safety (Healthcare Commission, 2006). Borrill et al. (2000) identified that staff working in teams within hospital-based care, reported lower levels of stress when compared to colleagues who worked alone or in less defined groupings. Moroney and Knowles (2006) similarly identified positive outcomes when they evaluated the implementation of multi-disciplinary team ward rounds; identifying an increase in patient involvement, a development of nurses and greater job satisfaction, and an improvement in MDT relationships, all of which improved ward culture and created a happier working environment.

Characteristics of effective teams

The 2005 *National Survey of NHS Staff* (Healthcare Commission, 2006) identified that 89 per cent of respondents reported that they work in a team, but for many groups of staff the teams appeared to be in name only and did not display all of the characteristics of a well-structured team. A well-structured team has been identified by the Healthcare Commission (2006) as having the following characteristics:

- The team objectives are clear.
- The team members work closely to achieve team objectives.

- Regular team meetings are held to discuss effectiveness and ways for improvement of the team.
- The team does not have more than 15 members.

Action point 10.3 – A well-structured team

Consider your clinical team in relation to the four characteristics identified by the Healthcare Commission as comprising a well-structured team. Does your team possess all of these characteristics? If the answer is no, you may wish to discuss your assessment with your manager and fellow team members.

Team roles

Belbin (1993) developed a theory, based on his research that individuals can contribute to team-working in a specific number of ways. He identified nine key team roles as outlined in Table 10.1. However, he also argues that not all nine roles are necessarily essential for the successful functioning of the team. Belbin also suggests that team members can display the qualities of more than one of the identified team roles. Belbin's research focused on management teams; however, the team roles are transferable to other types of teams.

Action point 10.4 – Team roles

Think about a team that you are a member of, and consider each of Belbin's team roles in turn. Make notes on which team role/s most closely represent your contribution to this team. Consider the remaining team roles – are these covered by the roles that your colleagues adopt within this team? Are there any roles that are not covered within the team? Do colleagues appear to adopt more than one role simultaneously? Now relating your reflections to the overall functioning of the team, consider how successful the team is. How do the dynamics of the team overcome some of the 'allowable weaknesses' identified in Belbin's identified team roles?

Multi-disciplinary team roles

Each of the disciplines that collectively comprise the multi-disciplinary team has their own professional values and code of conduct etc. Within nursing and midwifery, *The Code – Standards of Conduct, Performance and Ethics for Nurses and Midwives* (NMC, 2008a) outlines the requirement for the practitioner to 'work cooperatively within teams and respect the skills, expertise and contributions of your colleagues'. The NMC (2004a) *Standards of Proficiency for Pre-registration Nursing Education* similarly identifies standards for entry to the register that the practitioner is required to meet in relation to teamwork.

Table 10.1 *Team-Role Descriptions*

Team Role	Contribution	Allowable Weakness
Plant	Creative, imaginative, unorthodox. Solves difficult problems.	Ignores incidentals. Too pre-occupied to communicate effectively.
Resource Investigator	Extrovert, enthusiastic, communicative. Explores opportunities. Develops contacts.	Over-optimistic. Loses interest once initial enthusiasm has passed.
Co-ordinator	Mature, confident, a good chairperson. Clarifies goals, promotes decision-making, delegates well.	Can be seen as manipulative. Offloads personal work.
Shaper	Challenging, dynamic, thrives on pressure. The drive and courage to overcome obstacles.	Prone to provocation. Offends people's feelings.
Monitor Evaluator	Sober, strategic and discerning. Sees all options. Judges accurately.	Lacks drive and ability to inspire others.
Teamworker	Co-operative, mild, perceptive and diplomatic. Listens, builds, averts friction.	Indecisive in crunch situations.
Implementer	Disciplined, reliable, conservative and efficient. Turns ideas into practical actions.	Somewhat inflexible. Slow to respond to new possibilities.
Completer Finisher	Painstaking, conscientious, anxious. Searches out errors and omissions. Delivers on time.	Inclined to worry unduly. Reluctant to delegate.
Specialist	Single-minded, self-starting, dedicated. Provides knowledge and skills in rare supply.	Contributes on only a narrow front. Dwells on technicalities.

Source: Belbin (1993)

The role of the nurse in the multi-disciplinary team

Within the rehabilitation literature, a number of models have been developed that address the actual and potential role of the nurse in this area of practice. Hoeman (2002) for example discusses the care manager role of the nurse; and Lamb and Stempell (1994) make reference to the coordination role. These roles can be applied to other clinical specialties.

In *Modernising Nursing Careers: Setting the Direction,* the DH (2006c) identifies the future direction for nursing with regard to Government healthcare reforms. This report acknowledges that nurses do not work in isolation and need to lead the nursing workforce as part of multi-disciplinary teams. The report also highlights the need for nurses to have a 'sense of identity and confidence in their specific contribution to multidisciplinary teams'. In achieving the programme of healthcare reform, the report asserts that nursing careers need to move from nurses primarily engaged in care delivery to a model whereby they are additionally leaders, coordinators and commissioners of care (DH, 2006c).

Team leadership

Leadership can exist outside of formal hierarchical structures, and there is therefore a need to develop leaders at all levels within the organisation to facilitate both top-down and bottom-up approaches to development. In recent years the NHS has invested significantly in leadership education and development for its staff. The achievement of effective healthcare for patients requires the input of a number of management functions and professional groups across organisation. Some staff may work together in a collaborative function, while others may operate more as a team.

Leadership will now be explored within the context of teamwork. The leader should view fellow team members as partners and therefore having equality of status. This approach can facilitate a sharing of leadership amongst team members who are empowered to take a natural lead at times where they consider that they are in the best position to drive the team forward. The team needs to have vision and to collectively agree what it is aspiring to achieve. Effective leadership of the team is essential to ensure that it achieves its vision.

Challenges to leadership and management within inter-professional teams

Shared responsibility for outcomes is an integral feature of an inter-disciplinary team. This can present a challenge for the leader in managing accountability within shared responsibility. For some teams this may be further complicated by lack of clarity regarding team leadership. Within the inter-disciplinary team, individual members will have their lines of accountability and responsibility to their respective professional group that is often outside of the collective team.

A study conducted by Atwal and Caldwell (2006) regarding nurses' perceptions of teamwork in acute healthcare, identified three barriers that hindered teamwork: first, differing perceptions of teamwork; second, different levels of skills acquisitions to function as a team member; and third the dominance of medical power that influenced interaction in teams. Gibbon et al. (2002) identified that the introduction of team-coordinated approaches to stroke care and rehabilitation did not result in greater team-working staff attitudes.

Experiences of teamwork

A phenomenological study conducted by Robertson and Finlay (2007), revealed Occupational Therapists' relationships with multi-disciplinary colleagues to be both 'valuable and satisfying' while also providing a source of 'stress and frustration'. Team membership was valued by the Occupational Therapists both within their uni-disciplinary team and within the wider multi-disciplinary team. The Occupational

Therapists, however, considered that the extent of their role was misunderstood by colleagues, this being evidenced by colleagues focusing upon certain aspects of the role, such as the provision of equipment, to the exclusivity of others. A study by Saar and Trevizan (2007) similarly identified that participants in their study were not very knowledgeable about the professional roles of their colleagues. The role of the physician, nurse and pharmacist were found to be most understood, while the role of the psychologist was identified to be least understood.

 Action point 10.5 – Individual team members' roles

Refer back to the members of your team that you identified in Action point 10.1, and briefly outline the role of each member together with the unique contribution that this professional group brings to the inter-disciplinary team. Discuss your interpretations with individual team members. You may also find it helpful to explore the roles through the websites and literature that are published by the various professional bodies concerned.

Challenges to leadership and management within inter-agency teams

The challenges of team-working can be somewhat compounded within inter-agency teams; the membership, for example, comprises of staff from different organisations, each of which will have targets and outcomes to achieve that can sometimes conflict with one another. Acute hospitals, for example, need to meet waiting-time targets in accident and emergency departments and to reduce length of stay. Social care on the other hand is tasked with reducing reliance upon long-term institutional care and supporting independent living in the community. A focus on individual priorities, rather than a whole-systems approach, can be a cause of conflict between multi-agency team members. The joint appointment of a team leader across the agencies and professional disciplines, together with strong support and collective management, however, can maximise team performance.

Pooled budgets similarly present an opportunity to achieve more patient-centred services that span organisational boundaries. An example of an inter-agency team is a Hospital Discharge team that can include staff from social care, acute hospital care and primary care. The aim of such a team is to promote timely and seamless transfers of patient care from hospital back into the community. Benefits of this approach can include the minimising of duplication of effort, improved communication and maximising team performance. Furthermore, for teamwork to be effective, staff motivation is an important imperative, which is now explored.

Staff motivation

The DCM needs to be knowledgeable about the concept of motivation, together with the various approaches that managers can adopt on a day-to-day basis to motivate staff in order to maximise their effectiveness.

Why should the DCM be interested in staff motivation?

A few years ago, Brown (1998) suggested that national productivity could be raised 1.5 times if what was already known about motivation was implemented. Motivation had been shown to be the single most important factor in determining business (or work or organisation) efficiency. In concluding his views on staff motivation, Brown (1998:2) notes that 'Job satisfaction accounts for 25 per cent of the variation in productivity between organisations'; and goes on to suggest 'If you make people accountable as the drivers of the business rather than bit-part players, you have a direct impact on their motivation.'

It is important for the DCM to recognise the importance of motivation and its relevance to their role. Chapter 2 identified 'human resource manager' as one of 12 managerial roles of the DCM; the DCM needs to identify ways to motivate colleagues and subordinates in order to maximise productivity, develop individual and team spirit and to promote recruitment and retention.

Also as noted in Chapter 2, several definitions of management and manager refer to the activities and competencies of managers. Drucker (1979), for example, refers to management as working with and through individuals and groups to accomplish organisational goals. As this definition implies, managers are people to whom responsibility has been given, by virtue of the posts they are in, to ensure that the work of the organisation is carried out as specified in its strategic and operational plans. They have to decide the interventions that need to be performed, and suitable personnel to perform them. Rather than just telling employees which tasks to perform the manager needs to recognise that motivated staff will have a positive impact on productivity and quality.

 Action point 10.6 – Staff motivation in healthcare – an analysis

Consider the following questions and make notes in some detail:

- What motivates me to work?
- In what ways does my manager ensure that I remain motivated to do my work?
- How do I motivate my colleagues and subordinates?
- What else could managers/I do to motivate healthcare staff?

Motivation can be subdivided into two areas; *intrinsic* which is motivation from within, and *extrinsic* which is motivation by external rewards. Naturally one of the key reasons for working is to gain an income; other motivating factors include:

- Self-identity and a vocation
- Opportunity to engage in a subject area of interest
- Gaining new knowledge and skills
- An opportunity to help people – altruism
- Making friends.

Your manager may utilise a number of ways to motivate you and your colleagues at work, many of which can also be utilised by the DCM; these can include:

- supporting professional development;
- providing information, that is, knowledge of the reasons for new actions being taken;
- saying 'Thank you', 'Well done' at the end of a shift;
- setting adequately challenging tasks;
- encouraging and listening to ideas;
- identifying mutual goals through IDPRs;
- encouraging to use own initiative;
- encouraging social activities/outings;
- recognising high standards of care given, such as the absence of pressure sores and reduced re-admissions;
- allowing to introduce new ideas/methods of care (tested and untested); and
- being easily accessible, approachable and giving responsibility.

Many of the areas identified above also have relevance to the DCM role.

Theories of motivation

There are several theories of staff motivation documented in management literature. Different theories tend to apply to different circumstances and settings, and they may be combined by the user as appropriate. These theories include:

- Drucker's 'management by objectives'
- Maslow's theory of human motivation
- Herzberg on motivation to work
- McGregor's theory X and theory Y.

Management by objectives

One well recognised theory of staff motivation is Drucker's (1979) management by objectives (MBO). According to MBO, organisational goals (corporate objectives) are linked with employees' own personal needs and expectations of the job. A major point in MBO is that it directly attaches significance to individual employees' strengths and achievements at work rather than focusing on their weaknesses. MBO can be directly linked to IDPR.

Maslow's theory of human motivation

Maslow's (1987) theory of motivation is based upon the assumption that individuals are motivated to take action to fulfil particular human needs. Individuals strive to meet the more basic physiological needs first, and when this is satisfied they take action to meet their safety needs, then social needs, esteem needs, and finally their self-actualisation needs. Therefore, physical, safety and socio-economic needs have to be met first before the individual attempts to meet their higher psychological or intellectual needs and goals. However, Maslow suggested that if the self-actualisation or self-realisation needs of the individual are not satisfied, then problems of frustration, boredom and apathy might ensue.

Table 10.2 *Application of Maslow's theory of motivation to managing an organisation*

Needs level		Organisational rewards
1 *Physiological*	a)	Reasonable level of pay so that employees can easily afford, housing, food, clothing, etc.
	b)	Rest periods such as coffee breaks
	c)	A staff canteen
2 *Safety*	a)	Complying with health and safety regulations
	b)	Job security through employment contract and IDPR
	c)	Organisational policies, procedures and guidelines
3 *Social*	a)	Encouraging cohesive teamwork
	b)	Buddying and supportive supervision
	c)	Membership of sub teams
4 *Esteem*	a)	Acceptance of the individual by the team
	b)	Recognition of a job well done
5 *Self-actualisation*	a)	Preceptoring and clinical supervision
	b)	Opportunities to use initiative and creativity
	c)	Staff development strategies
	d)	Opportunities for advancement and career progression

However, meeting physiological needs does not present a problem to most individuals, and therefore they are more motivated to achieve or sustain their next level needs in the hierarchy. Several individuals knowingly jeopardise lower level needs in the quest for higher level needs of self-esteem and self-fulfilment, and therefore people's major needs centre around realising their full potential as individuals, via creative, worthwhile achievement. As a means of staff motivation, employing organisations and managers should endeavour to meet employees' needs as identified in Table 10.2.

Herzberg's theory of motivation to work

Modern theories of motivation are based on preceding theories and the findings of earlier experiments. Herzberg's theory on 'motivation to work' reflects the findings of the Hawthorne experiments conducted in the earlier part of the last century. The conclusions of the Hawthorne experiments indicated that productivity increases if individuals have stability, a place where they feel they belong, work in groups, and the purpose of the work is communicated to them.

Herzberg (1974) also suggested that all attempts to motivate employees by fear, economic rewards and good working conditions achieve limited success. In his view the way to motivate employees (which he considers to be intrinsic) is that in addition to providing the economic rewards and good working conditions, employees should simultaneously be given challenging work for which they can assume responsibility and gain the satisfaction of achievement.

Herzberg identified 'motivators or growth factors' by which employees are motivated, namely: a sense of achievement, recognition, responsibility and opportunities for personal growth and advancement. In addition to motivators, employers need to address the 'dissatisfiers' at work, which are also referred to as 'hygiene or maintenance factors'. These factors are:

- The level of supervision
- Interpersonal relations
- Working conditions
- Salary
- Company policies
- Administrative practices
- Job security.

McGregor's theory X and theory Y

McGregor (1987) suggests that false assumptions about human motivation lie at the root of many ineffective management strategies. He postulated that either 'theory X' or 'theory Y' about human nature and human behaviour formed the basis for every managerial decision or action. Thus managers who act in accordance with the principles of theory X tend to believe the following to be true of people and therefore their employees – that the average human being:

- has an inherent dislike of work and will avoid it if he can;
- prefers to be directed, wishes to avoid responsibility, has relatively little ambition and wants security above all; and
- must be coerced, controlled, directed and threatened with punishment to get them to put forth adequate effort towards the achievement of organisational objectives.

The assumption underpinning theory X is that most workers are interested in their work to only a limited extent, and therefore need to be coerced and threatened to ensure they carry out their duties effectively. Theory X offers management an easy rationalisation for ineffective organisational performance. McGregor's 'theory Y' is the polarised extreme of 'theory X', which reflects a more realistic assumption that recognises the importance of the individual's need for self-actualisation at work. The manager using theory Y tends to believe that for the average human being, and therefore their employees – that they:

- do not inherently dislike work;
- will exercise self-direction and self-control in the service of objectives to which they are committed;
- have commitment to organisational objectives as a function of the rewards associated with their achievement;
- learn under the appropriate conditions, not only to accept but also to seek responsibility;
- have capacity to exercise a relatively high degree of imagination, ingenuity and creativity in the solution of organisational problems;
- only partially utilise the intellectual abilities of their individual employees.

Theory Y reflects different implications for managerial strategy than those of theory X. It is dynamic rather than static, and recognises the opportunities for personal growth and development of employees. It enables managers to view their employees as resources, with substantial potentialities, and endeavour to enable them to discover how to realise their potential through its human resources department. These assumptions are apparent in managerial policies and practices.

Inter-professional team-working

Inter-professional learning has been advocated as a mechanism to promote inter-professional working. Empirical evidence to support such approaches, however, is limited and as such appears to be premised upon the rationale that if the various professional groups are expected to work together in teams then it is commonsensical to mirror this within educational preparation. A systematic review of the literature on evaluations of inter-professional education conducted by Freeth et al. (2002) identified that studies were predominantly focused on post-registration education in hospital or community-based service delivery settings, rather than those provided within academic institutions. The professional groups most represented were nursing and medicine, and the education was found to relate to two main categories, namely, traditional staff development, or that provided in response to an identified service development need.

Caldwell et al. (2006) conducted a study that explored pre-registration education in relation to teamwork, together with the perceptions of newly qualified practitioners regarding their confidence in working as a team member. The study identified overall positive reporting by respondents regarding their teamwork, with the exception of 'equality' where 47 per cent of respondents rated that they were either unsure or disagreed with the statement 'I have found that within my team the members work as equals'. The findings of Caldwell et al. are encouraging and would appear to support inter-professional education within pre-registration preparation; more research is needed, however, to evaluate the outcomes of such educational strategies in assessing both collective experiences and those of the respective professional disciplines.

Barr (2002) completed a systematic review of the literature regarding inter-professional education and argues that to be effective, inter-professional education must reflect the following areas.

1	*Put service users at the centre:*	Involving patients and clients in designing, teaching, participating and assessing programmes.
2	*Promote collaboration:*	Applying learning to collaborative practice during placements or work-based assignments, collaboration within and between professions, within and between organisations and with communities, service users and their carers.
3	*Reconcile competing objectives:*	Ensure that these principles are protected as the essential qualities of inter-professional education while ensuring that they are compatible with other objectives and

their implications for programme design, content and learning methods.

4 *Reinforce collaborative competence:* Reach beyond modification of attitudes and securing common knowledge bases to reinforce collaborative competencies necessary to cope with the complexity of contemporary practice.

5 *Relate collaboration in learning and practice to a coherent rationale:* for example, able to explain the beneficial outcomes of inter-professional learning.

6 *Incorporate inter-professional values:* for example, inclusion, equality, openness, humility, mutuality, generosity and reciprocity.

7 *Include common and comparative learning:* Treat comparative content as essential to inform learning from and about each other, to enhance understanding about respective roles and responsibilities and intelligent co-working.

8 *Employ a repertoire of interactive learning methods:* Avoid over-reliance on any one method.

9 *Count towards qualifications:* Inter-professional education is valued more when it is assessed towards qualifications.

10 *Assess and evaluate programmes:* It is also valued more when programmes are approved and, where feasible, evaluated.

11 *Disseminate findings:* To inform, stimulate and support wider development of inter-professional education.

Leadership, power and hierarchies

Inter-professional teamwork also requires leadership, although in healthcare it has traditionally been perceived as hierarchical in nature and defined by job title and position equating to the status of the individual within the organisation. Snelgrove and Hughes (2002) conducted interviews with medical and nursing staff in three general hospitals; their study identified that teamwork was seen to be valuable by both professional groups; however, the 'power of medical hierarchies and the limits of nursing influence in core areas of medical work' was recognised. The concept power relates to control, influence and authority and can be subdivided into various cognate areas as identified in Box 3.4 in Chapter 3.

The NHS Leadership Qualities Framework (NHS III, 2006) identifies 15 leadership qualities that include personal, cognitive and social qualities that are applicable to leadership roles at all levels within the health service, both existing and aspiring. The leadership qualities are arranged in three clusters – Personal Qualities, Setting Direction, and Delivering the Service. For each individual quality there are between three and six levels, each of which commences with a negative descriptor that describes behaviours that illustrate a lack of the individual quality. Collaborative working is one of the five qualities that feature within the 'Delivering the Service' cluster. The other four qualities include leading change through people, holding to account, empowering others and effective and strategic influencing.

Action point 10.7 – Levels of working

Consider your interrelationships with key stakeholders, including patients, carers, health professionals, social care professionals together with voluntary sector organisations. For each stakeholder identified, consider which collaborative level from the following provided by the NHS Institute for Innovation and Improvement (2006), best describes your current level of working.

0. *Goes it alone*	
• Fails to involve others in bringing about integrated healthcare.	Yes/No
• Does not share information with other stakeholders.	Yes/No
1. *Appreciates others' views*	
• Expresses positive expectations of internal and external stakeholders.	Yes/No
• Acknowledges and respects others' diverse perspectives.	Yes/No
2. *Works for shared understanding*	
• Shares information with partners when appropriate.	Yes/No
• Summarises progress, taking account of differing viewpoints, so as to clarify understanding and to establish common ground.	Yes/No
• Surfaces conflict and supports resolution of this conflict.	Yes/No
3. *Forges partnerships for the long term*	
• Works with other stakeholders where conflict impedes progress to create the conditions for successful partnership working in the longer term.	Yes/No
• Is informed on the current priorities of partners, and responds appropriately to changes in their status or circumstances.	Yes/No
• Ensures that the strategy for health improvement is developed in a cohesive and 'joined up' manner.	Yes/No

Source: NHS Institute for Innovation and Improvement (2006)

You may wish to consider completing a more comprehensive self-assessment by addressing all of the qualities that are included within the Leadership Qualities Framework. Now develop a personal action plan that includes strategies for you to further develop your collaborative working. You may find it helpful to discuss this with your manager, mentor or preceptor, as appropriate.

Communication

Teams need to have effective communication to enable them to achieve their goals. Communication is central to sharing information and to the facilitation of group problem-solving and decision-making. We communicate using a combination of verbal and non-verbal approaches. Verbal communication encompasses the words that we say, together with the way in which we say them. Non-verbal communication relates to the messages that we provide to other people through our body language, as discussed in Chapter 1. In addition to face-to-face communication, a number of other strategies are also available to support communication with members of the inter-disciplinary team such as telephone, paper and electronic formats.

It should be borne in mind that communication encompasses much more than simply sending a message. Communication is a two-way process, the success of which is dependent upon the receiver interpreting the information in the way that the sender had intended. Messages sent electronically, for example, can be left open to interpretation by the receiver as they are unable to establish the tone in which the message has been sent.

The *Essence of Care* (DH, 2003) includes benchmarks for communication between patients, carers and healthcare personnel. Factor Eight focuses on the coordination of care, for which the identified benchmark of best practice is stated 'all care providers communicate fully and effectively with each other to ensure that patients' and/or carers' benefit from a comprehensive plan of care which is regularly updated and evaluated'. As with all of the benchmarks, the communication benchmark includes indicators of best practice that have been developed by patients, carers and professionals to support the achievement of best practice.

 Action point 10.8 – Communication benchmarks

Some of the indicators of best practice that are included as part of the communication benchmarks (DH, 2003) are identified below. For each of the indicators listed, complete a self-assessment regarding how your practice setting measures up. You may find it helpful to discuss some of the indicators with patients, carers and colleagues to establish their perspectives.

1	Patients and or carers who are physically isolated or unable to communicate directly with significant others are enabled to communicate.	Yes/No
2	Patients and or carers have choice about where they exchange information.	Yes/No

3	Restrictions to communication are explained.	Yes/No
4	Assessment of the needs of patients and or carers identifies where and when communication should take place.	Yes/No
5	The inclusion of other people when communication occurs is agreed with the patients and or carers.	Yes/No
6	There is an appropriately furnished, separate and specially designated room.	Yes/No
7	The environment is inclusive and adapted to meet differing communication needs in terms of, for example, lighting, acoustic conditions, hearing loops.	Yes/No
8	The environment supports communication and audit of the environment, including signage and maps to present information.	Yes/No
9	Appointment times are arranged to facilitate communication.	Yes/No
10	Mechanisms are in place to ensure necessary follow-up appointments are made.	Yes/No
11	Advocacy services are engaged according to the wishes of patients and/or carers.	Yes/No
12	Patients and or carers are identified in order to discuss treatment and care, when face-to-face communication is not possible, for example, by using a Password system.	Yes/No
13	Communication between patients and or carers and health care personnel is recorded.	Yes / No

Adapted from: *Essence of Care* (DH, 2003:41).

Once you have completed this action point, compare the results for the various groups that you have consulted, and consider whether you can identify any discrepancies, or whether the results were consistent across all groups. For the indicators for which you have identified a 'no' response, you may find it helpful to discuss with your manager and members of your team to establish why this area of best practice has not been implemented. Are there any plans to address this? Could it be a shared objective for the team? If so, are there any other stakeholders who would need to be involved?

Poor communication is often identified as a key contributing factor in the investigation of complaints about health services. The Parliamentary and Health Service Ombudsman report (2006), for example, identified poor communication between patients and carers, and lack of 'essential communication' and coordination between services as examples of poor practice that illustrate a lack of patient focus. Such features were further reported as being more prevalent in complaints relating to older people, together with people who have a mental illness.

Strategies to support multi-professional communication

Team meetings are essential to ensure effective communication between team members. The team may engage in various meetings together, each of which should fulfil a different function. These can include meetings to discuss patient progress and to set patient goals; together with meetings to maximise the effectiveness of the team, for instance, where team goals are set and outcomes are monitored.

Getting the most out of group/team meetings

Meetings need to be managed effectively to ensure that they are productive and meet the needs of the team and its members. As the DCM, in addition to being a team member, you may also find yourself in the position of leading a group/team meeting; this could be for a handover report to colleagues, or for discussing your patients as part of a multi-disciplinary team meeting. To maximise the outcomes of these meetings, there are a number of principles that should be adhered to, as follows:

- Always start and finish the meeting on time.
- Review progress achieved since the last meeting.
- Encourage all members to participate.
- Keep focused on the nature of the business.
- Summarise key points.
- Agree the outcomes to be achieved by the next meeting.
- Confirm date and time of next meeting.

In addition to face-to-face communication, the multi-disciplinary team needs to ensure effective record-keeping, both as a formal record of the care provided, together with providing a mechanism to share information. Traditional record-keeping systems maintained by each discipline are not conducive to teamwork and can lead to duplication of effort. Therapists for example may maintain their discipline-specific records and additionally record a brief summary of interventions and treatments in the patient's notes. Integrated record-keeping systems can be more conducive to teamwork, as they contain a comprehensive account of the interventions of each member of the multi-disciplinary team. The Single Assessment Process (SAP), as outlined in Chapter 9, provides an example of an integrated record that can be multi-professional and multi-agency, and can also be utilised as a patient-held record.

NHS Connecting for Health (CfH) aims to support the NHS to deliver better and safer care to patients; through IT systems that link GPs and community services to hospitals. The NHS Care Records Service (NHS CRS) forms part of the work of CfH, and links patient information from different parts of the NHS electronically. Information relating to the benefits of the NHS CRS can be found by accessing the CfH website: http://www.connectingforhealth.nhs.uk/. The aim of this work is to ensure that NHS staff and patients have access to the information that they require to support care and treatment decisions.

Ineffective teamwork

Whilst the various merits of teamwork are espoused and this model of working is widely promoted, it must be recognised that not all teams are effective. The report of the public inquiry into children's heart surgery at the British Royal Infirmary between 1984 and 1995 (Kennedy, 2001), for example, cited failings in communication together with a lack of leadership and teamwork as a contributing factor for the failings. A clear lack of clinical leadership was identified as being responsible for the poor teamwork that was in existence. This report made a number of recommendations that included the need for managers, doctors and nurses to work together and to have clear lines of accountability.

As identified in Chapter 4, conflict can provide a source of challenge for groups and teams. To facilitate effective teamwork, individual team members need to have clarity regarding their personal role, together with the roles of their fellow team members. The language used by team members can provide insight into team cohesiveness, language such as 'we' and 'us', for example, suggests ownership and a unified approach.

 Action point 10.9 – Effective teams and ineffective teams

First, consider a successful team that you have been a member of. Make notes on what the characteristics were that made the team a success. What skills and attributes did the leader of the team demonstrate?

Second, consider a less effective team that you have been a member of. Why was this team less effective? How did the skills and attributes of the leader differ to those of the more effective leader in the successful team that you identified?

Evaluating team performance

Throughout the chapter, reference has been made to the numerous challenges associated with teamwork. Within healthcare there is a need to maximise the use of resources and to ensure best outcomes for patients.

Measures that can be utilised to measure the effectiveness of teamwork can include:

- Patient outcomes – for example, functional independence, independent living, quality of life
- Service efficiency – for example, length of stay, service costs
- Patient satisfaction – for example, communication, seamless transfer of care.

In order to evaluate the effectiveness of a team it is helpful to have clarity of purpose that can be used as a benchmark against which to assess team performance. First, it is helpful to establish if the team has:

- a mission statement that articulates shared purpose and values;
- shared goals; and
- agreed SMART objectives.

SMART is an acronym for **S**pecific, **M**easurable, **A**chievable, **R**ealistic and **T**imed. It is worth exploring how recently the mission statement, goals and objectives have been reviewed to ensure clarity and focus for the team. Mechanisms to appraise team performance should also be agreed.

 Action point 10.10 – The successful team

Think about your team, how effective do you consider it to be? What has the team achieved during the past 12 months? What strategies, both formal and informal are utilised to provide both the whole team and individual members with feedback? You may find it beneficial to ask members of your team the same questions and to explore with your manager and as a team how you can further enhance team-working and maximise outcomes.

Celebrating and sharing success

When the team evaluates its performance against the goals that it had set, it is important to make it a priority to both celebrate and share its achievements. There are a number of ways that this can be achieved: for example, organising a team celebration or night out; informing managers of the accomplishments; submitting an abstract to present a paper at a conference, writing an article for publication in a professional journal and submitting an application for an award.

Guidelines for coherent and effective inter-professional teamwork

The following, constitute good practice guidelines for coherent and effective inter-professional teamwork.

- Ensure that the patient is the focus of your teamwork.
- As a team, develop and agree your mission statement and goals.
- Set SMART objectives.
- Ensure that your team and its objectives support the wider organisation.
- Agree how you will communicate with team members and the wider organisation.
- Monitor team performance and evaluate outcomes.
- Celebrate and share team success.

Chapter summary

Teamwork is premised as an important mechanism for healthcare management and delivery. Whether uni-disciplinary, inter-disciplinary or inter-agency, the team needs to have clarity of purpose, together with clear objectives to enable it to be effective. Individual teams also need to operate within the overarching objectives of the wider organisation. Effective teamwork is dependant upon good working relationships and effective communication between team members. The DCM has an important role in coordinating uni-disciplinary, inter-disciplinary and inter-agency care and the needs of the patient should be central to the focus of such teamwork.

This chapter has focused on uni-professional, inter-professional and inter-agency teamwork in healthcare and therefore focused on:

- theories of teamwork, which entailed differentiation between groups and teams, identifying models and benefits of teamwork, the characteristics of effective teams and multi-disciplinary team roles, including the role of the nurse in the multi-disciplinary team;
- team leadership, including experiences of teamwork, challenges to leadership and management within inter-professional teams and within inter-agency teams;
- staff motivation, which started by exploring why the DCM should have knowledge and understanding of staff motivation, what motivation is, theories of motivation such as management by objectives, Maslow's theory of human motivation based on human needs, Herzberg's theory comprising motivators and hygiene factors and McGregor's theory X and theory Y with regards to how employees are perceived by managers; and
- inter-professional education, which included exploring power and hierarchies within and between healthcare professions, multi-professional communication and strategies to ensure they are effective, getting the most out of inter-professional team meetings, ineffective teamwork, evaluation of team performance and guidelines for coherent and effective inter-professional teamwork.

ELEVEN Managing learning in practice settings

Introduction

Organisations proudly and strategically display Investors in People (IIP) shields and use the logo on their organisations' headed paper to indicate that both employees and employers value ongoing learning. Continuing professional development (CPD) and lifelong learning are also essential activities under the clinical governance framework, which in turn enriches the learning ethos in practice settings. Such environments encourage and invest in formal modes of learning, and also support informal learning activities. Informal learning generally refers to various non-structured learning and teaching that healthcare organisations quiescently support. This chapter analyses the way in which a learning ethos can prevail in practice settings, and thereby ensure that employees and patients benefit from up-to-date knowledge and competence. It examines how learning in practice settings is managed, with the ultimate aim of ensuring safe and effective care delivery.

Chapter objectives

On completion of this chapter you will be able to:

- identify the ways in which the healthcare registrant progresses from being a preceptee through to functioning competently as a DCM, and beyond;
- demonstrate knowledge of what makes practice settings learning environments, and how the DCM manages and sustains a learning ethos in these settings;
- demonstrate substantial insight into how the DCM can influence an organisational culture that values and supports learning;
- suggest how to utilise and maximise opportunities for the acquisition of knowledge and professional competence in the development and education of healthcare practitioners; and
- recognise developmental processes that incorporate CPD, lifelong learning, professional regulation and funding for CPD.

Progressing from registrant to DCM

Practice settings that are effective learning environments are those that enable the professional and personal development of healthcare practitioners. It involves supporting learning for everyone, including those who are on structured courses and those who are not, and includes mentoring, preceptorship and supervision. It also includes identifying and developing learning opportunities for all healthcare profession students and learners. Mentoring in healthcare, which is also known by various other titles such as practice supervision and clinical education and tends to refer to facilitation of learning for pre-registration students, and preceptoring refers to facilitation of learning for new registrants. Learning beyond preceptoring includes management coaching. Peer support and learning for qualified staff were discussed under clinical supervision and peer review in Chapter 8.

Being a preceptee

On first qualifying and registering with the appropriate professional regulatory body, the registrant undergoes a period of preceptorship, which involves supervised practice for a specified but flexible length of time. Starting a first job as a qualified practitioner can be both exciting and daunting.

 Action point 11.1 – Hopes, fears and solutions of finalist healthcare students

Consider the hopes and fears of emerging healthcare practitioners at the point of registration, and jot these down together with some of the possible reasons for these, and potential solutions.

Various hopes and fears are experienced by new registrants when they seek employment on qualifying. Some of the hopes and fears of aspiring healthcare practitioners are identified on Table 11.1.

Table 11.1 *Hopes and fears of aspiring healthcare practitioners*

Hopes	Fears
• Acceptance and support from staff	• Isolation (lack of support) due to staff shortages
• Orientation to the clinical environment and systems	• Not fitting into the MDT
• Space for gaining experience and confidence	• Personal expectations not being met
• Support for further professional education	• Not being valued
• An identified preceptorship period, and clinical supervision	• Making mistakes
• To learn how to practise safely and effectively	• Personality clashes
• A Band 5 development programme	• Aggressive patients/staff
• To further develop clinical skills	• Anxiety due to lack of confidence in own competence, and fear of litigation
• Equal opportunities for all team members	• Insufficient professional development time
• To be valued as an important member of the clinical team	• Dealing with complaints – due to lack of experience

As can be expected, new registrants' hopes vary from individual to individual. Some of the ways in which fears can be prevented from materialising are as follows. For fear of isolation (lack of support) due to staff shortages, or of making mistakes for instance, the registrants need to invest full effort into their day-to-day clinical interventions, look for role models and observe experienced colleagues. They must support their activities through further reading and attending appropriate structured learning events. Access to structured preceptorship can play a crucial role. For personality clashes, they would need to learn how to resolve this experientially; it may help to discuss this with the preceptor, and also attend assertiveness training. For overcoming inexperience and lack of self-confidence in dealing with complaints, the registrant needs to become fully conversant with appropriate policies and procedures, which include documentation, and accessing relevant departments in the organisation.

Several authorities, including the NMC (2006c), indicate that the support and guidance of an experienced professional colleague can be invaluable for a newly registered healthcare practitioner, for a registrant who has returned to practice following a break of five years or more, or for a registrant changing their area of practice, and for qualified nurses from other European Economic Area States and overseas. The provision of such support and guidance is referred to as preceptorship, and has been recommended for some time as a form of formal support that incorporates learning time that is protected during the first year of qualified practice, depending on preceptee's ability and experience.

The preceptor's role has different meanings in different professions, and even in nursing in different countries. In England and Wales, preceptorship refers to a specified but negotiable period of structured support and facilitation of learning for registrants who are new to the specialism, to consolidate existing skills and theoretical knowledge, and to develop new skills that are required for the specialism.

Preceptoring aims to reduce the phenomenon of *Reality Shock* (Kramer, 1974; Bain, 1996) that can occur on transition from being a mentored student to an accountable practitioner, and characterised by initial period of disorientation. Therefore, preceptorship prepares newly qualified healthcare practitioners for responsible and accountable professional practice and protects the public from the inexperienced. It also initiates socialisation of the newly qualified healthcare practitioners into the team and its routines, and can lead to higher morale and better retention and recruitment of staff.

The NMC notes that preceptors will not, however, be accountable for the actions or omissions of preceptees, as they are registered practitioners and therefore accountable for their practice. Preceptorship is not a mandatory requirement and the NMC has no power to enforce the system, but it emphatically states that structured preceptorship reflects sound professional practice, and advise that local policies should be developed or amended for this purpose. The NMC's (2006c) recommendations for preceptors are that they should:

- facilitate the transition from student to a registrant who is: confident in his/her practice, sensitive to the needs of patients, an effective team member and up-to-date with their practice and knowledge;
- provide feedback to new registrants on good performance;

- provide honest, constructive and objective feedback on performance that needs improvement and provide support to remedy this; and
- facilitate new registrants to gain new knowledge and skills.

It constitutes an intensive but short-term teaching and supervisory role. A preceptor is therefore a person, generally a staff nurse (in the nursing profession), who teaches, counsels, inspires, serves as a role model and supports the professional growth and development of an individual (the novice) for a fixed period of time with the specific purpose of enabling skill development and socialising the novice into the new role.

The NMC (2006c) also indicates that healthcare practitioners who take on the role of preceptor should be first level registrants who have had at least 12 months (or equivalent) experience within the same area of practice as the registrant requiring support. Registrants may be in full or part-time employment, but they must appreciate the additional demands it places upon them, and have appropriate preparation for the role. The preceptor and the preceptee should agree the nature of their working relationship and define intended outcomes, which at times comprise an adaptation of the induction programme for new employees, and can be documented as a learning contract. Midwives also have the support of a named supervisor of midwives allocated upon starting to practise midwifery.

Preceptors can be called upon if the registrant needs help with a procedure that they are unfamiliar with, or with a situation not encountered before, or if guidance is needed with certain aspect of practice. However, there can be barriers to effective functioning of the preceptorship role, which can include poor staffing levels, lack of time to precept and lack of baseline criteria to measure progress against.

As to the preparation of preceptors, structured preceptorship programmes can be provided locally by employing organisations. There are no formal qualifications associated with being a preceptor, but preparation as a mentor or practice teacher should provide a sound basis for anyone undertaking the role.

Management coaching for the DCM

Taken from the viewpoint that healthcare practitioners' functions can be grouped under key areas such as the six core dimensions (or components) stipulated in the *NHS KSF* (DH, 2004a), these components are learnt under both mentoring and preceptoring provision as just discussed.

Government policies such as the *NHS KSF* (DH, 2004a), have relevance for the DCM's role. This framework of job definitions for healthcare employees identifies posts into pay bands, and also provides a basis for review and development. The IDPR is designed to (DH, 2004a):

- identify the knowledge and skills that individuals need to apply in their post;
- help to guide the development of individuals;
- provide a fair and objective framework on which to base review and development for all staff; and
- provide the basis of pay progression in the service.

The *NHS KSF* and the accompanying process has been developed through a partnership approach between management and staff representatives. This partnership approach is intended to continue as the *NHS KSF* is used in development review, with managers working with individual members of staff to plan their training and development and review their work. Thereby, one of the key principles on which the *NHS KSF* is based is that of identifying a competence framework that should be able to support the ongoing development of the NHS itself.

Teaching skills can be learnt through both pre-registration and mentoring courses, and the teaching role of the registrant is clearly identified by the NMC (2008b) and other professional bodies. Research skills can be acquired through attending specific courses, journal clubs, completing assignments and conducting research under the guidance of a supervisor. How then are management skills learned?

Attending management courses is one way to learn management skills. Some insight into aspects of management will have been gained through pre-registration programmes, particularly during the final practice placement. However, to a substantial extent, management skills are acquired through work-based experiences in the practice setting.

 Action point 11.2 – How the DCM learns management skills

Consider from your own experiences how DCMs learn the management skills as an inherent component of their jobs. Consider healthcare practitioners on band 5 or 6 who you know, and reflect on how they acquired their management skills.

In addition to experiential learning, DCMs as first level managers often learn management skills from their line or more senior managers. Work-based learning theories, which are discussed shortly significantly underpin this. Management coaching is another systematic means of acquiring management skills.

As a term that is generally used in sports and general physical fitness, as well as in management training, coaching tends to refer to one-to-one and team guidance in developing or improving skills and performance. Driscoll and Cooper (2005) suggest that it is a holistic term for the support of continuing personal and professional development. This function includes enabling the coachee to reflect on, and to draw their own conclusions about the best way to develop and enhance their skills. This applies to the DCM as a developing manager as they are both empowered and accountable for their management functions. This form of learning can comprise regular one-to-one meetings between the DCM and the coach, supported by structured study days.

Various management skills were identified in Chapter 2, Table 2.1, as day-to-day management activities of the DCM. It is important, of course, for the coach to be competent in both coaching and management skills. An alternative to the management coach can be a mentor to the trainee manager. Fields (1994) suggest that if a mentoring relationship is used instead of a coach, then the management mentor should be a more senior and experienced manager, but not in a line management relationship with the mentee. They could be from a different part of the organisation, or even external to the organisation.

Here a clear distinction is being made between a management coach and a management mentor. The definition of a mentor would in this case be different to the NMC (2008b) definition which specifically refers to facilitation of learning and assessment of competence. Instead, as Byrne and Keefe' (2002) suggest, the mentor is a person who helps a more junior person develop professionally through a combination of advising, skill development, creation of opportunities and personal growth in an intense manner over an extended period of time. Fields (1994) suggests that typically the management mentor should be chosen by the trainee manager, with the knowledge that the mentor has certain specific qualities or attributes that are desirable. It is also preferable for the mentor to have undertaken educational preparation for the role.

Driscoll and Cooper (2005) differentiate between clinical supervision and management coaching, and note that while the former is still viewed with suspicion by supervisees and is often difficult to implement due to lack of time, the latter is already available to some senior managers in healthcare, whereupon individually tailored personal and professional development meetings intended to improve organisational performance are held. Gould et al. (2001) report on a study exploring nurse managers' perceptions of factors that help or hinder their performance, in which the latter reported poor preparation to undertake key aspects of their roles. Educational preparation for management roles can be accessed in various ways such as in-service courses, and open learning programmes such as the Master of Business Administration courses offered by some higher education institutes.

Supervising learning

Supervision of healthcare students and learners is an important role of the DCM. The various learners and healthcare students whose learning needs to be facilitated in the practice setting can include CSWs on national vocational qualification courses, and nursing, medical and AHP students. Mentoring refers to enabling pre-registration students to develop clinical skills. The NMC (2008b) has identified competencies and outcomes for mentors that the mentor has to achieve through professional preparation to be competent to practise as a mentor. The mentoring role usually incorporates the assessment of learners competence (e.g. ENB/DH, 2001; NMC, 2008b), and recording them in appropriate documents. Gopee (2008) identifies various approaches and models of mentoring. These can include one-to-one and team mentoring, with a named mentor being allocated to a student (or the student selecting their own mentor). Some students might select a mentor in each placement; others might also negotiate with one individual to whom they could relate throughout the entire programme. The role will imminently develop to the sign-off mentor role whose function will include assessing finalist students on an identified set of clinical skills to ensure they are 'fit for practice'.

A similar arrangement can apply to preceptorship which refers to supervising learning for newly qualified healthcare practitioners. There are common elements and differences between mentoring and preceptoring, but the principles of facilitation of learning for qualified staff, that is, preceptoring are similar to those of mentoring, and it is generally expected that the preceptor already holds a mentor qualification (NMC, 2008b).

Action point 11.3 – Allocating mentors and preceptors

How are mentors and preceptors allocated to learners in your practice setting? Explore, and decide whether you have any views on how they can be allocated more effectively.

The NMC (2006c, 2008b) indicate that both roles require identifying a named person, but one who is supported by team members.

Enhancing the practice setting as a learning environment

It is the responsibility of the DCM to supervise and monitor the practice of all individuals in the workforce so that competent, safe and effective care is delivered at all times. Individual employees also have the responsibility to ensure they acknowledge any limitations in their knowledge and skills and are open to develop new knowledge and skills. To achieve this, an enquiring open-minded trusting ethos in the workplace is essential. This section explores this aspect of practice settings, and includes healthcare professionalism and CPD, the care setting as a learning environment, work-based or practice-based learning, practice settings as learning organisations and organisational culture.

Professionalism and CPD

It is every healthcare practitioner's responsibility, to engage in CPD, a concept which is a subset of lifelong learning (DH, 2001c; Gopee, 2001). This is to ensure that their clinical practice is informed by current knowledge and evidence. As noted in Chapter 8, this is achieved through formal and non-formal processes, that is, through attending structured courses, or more informal training and education. Non-formal learning refers to structured teaching and learning strategies that do not involve attending structured courses. It therefore includes short courses held in the health-care trust's post-graduate or in-service training department. Each trust has staff development strategies in their annual business plans. They work in tandem with IDPRs and personal development plans as indicated in the *NHS KSF* (DH, 2004a).

Furthermore, substantial learning of knowledge and competence occurs while engaging in direct patient care, hence the concept work-based learning. It is logical to deduce therefore that the patient-care setting and general work ethos should reflect an environment where learning is fostered and supported. Teaching and learning, that is, facilitating the acquisition of knowledge and competence in practice settings, is also a feature of professionalism, as indicated in the NMC (2008a) *The Code – Standards of Conduct, Performance and Ethics for Nurses and Midwives*, for instance. However, such learning can also be referred to as 'incidental learning', which can be seen positively as 'opportunistic' learning, or with reservation as unstructured and partial learning.

*Continuing professional development and
lifelong learning*

To avoid waiting for opportunities to learn, the healthcare practitioner can endeavour to be more proactive, anticipate problematic situations and encounter them as natural challenges. This tends to implicate ongoing learning. Various policy documents including *The PREP Handbook* (NMC, 2006b), *Working Together, Learning Together* (DH, 2001c), *Continuing Professional Development* (GMC, 2004) recognise the importance of CPD and lifelong learning for all throughout our professional careers. Clinical supervision, as just discussed, is one formal medium through which individuals can identify their professional development needs; IDPR is another. More informal means of support and identifying professional development needs include peer-assessment (and peer-review), together with social capital; as discussed in Chapter 8.

Furthermore, as noted in Chapter 7, Handy (1984) suggests that people should be treated as assets, not costs and that the workplace has a vital role to play in fostering continuing learning. Thus, as lifelong learning is becoming increasingly appreciated as an essential ingredient for ensuring high quality patient care, it would seem that employers and employees need to be sensitive to and nurture all structures that can facilitate this. Apart from the organisational mechanisms that are in situ to facilitate CPD for healthcare practitioners, informal learning tends to go unrecognised or is under-utilised, as also noted in Chapter 8.

Learning opportunities for healthcare practitioners

Numerous avenues of learning have developed during the last two decades. Professional development courses run at universities and short courses in healthcare trusts own in-service/post-graduate training departments constitute the majority of professional development provision. Others include:

- structured teaching by medical staff, clinical nurse specialists and practice facilitators, for instance;
- conferences organised locally by healthcare trusts;
- conferences organised by professional forums;
- e-learning or blended learning opportunities;
- professional development learning and assessment provision in professional journals; and
- inter-professional learning.

In the current ethos of efficiency, effectiveness and targets for healthcare delivery, teaching and learning can easily be relegated to being a fringe activity. Therefore DCMs should ensure that opportunities for the acquisition of knowledge and competencies are maximised. Such opportunities could comprise use of e-learning and blended learning that can be accessed from practice settings.

The practice setting as a learning environment

Nursing is a practice-based profession and a substantial part of learning that the 'novice' nurse undertakes occurs in the practice setting.

Action point 11.4 – The practice setting as a learning environment

Reflect on your experiences of the various practice settings where you have worked. Consider the question 'what makes a care and treatment setting a learning environment?' Think of the settings where you or learners have had a positive learning experience and contrast them with those where learning is less well supported.

The NMC (2008b: 53) identifies a learning environment as one 'where practice is valued and developed, that provides appropriate professional and inter-professional learning opportunities and support for learning to maximise achievement for individuals'. It refers to a range of practice settings including hospital wards, health centres and schools, which self-evidently constitute important learning environments.

Dunn and Hansford (1997) note that a clinical learning environment comprises an interactive network of forces that influence student learning outcomes in practice settings. These descriptions implicitly recognise the psycho-social factors that are essential for practice settings to be learning environments, and therefore Gopee (2008) concludes that a practice setting that constitutes a learning environment comprises a psycho-social ethos and culture with related supportive resources that foster mutual learning amongst all stakeholder healthcare practitioners, learners and clientele, and where care and treatment are founded on evidence-based practice. Stuart (2007) suggests that there are four categories of factors that make a practice setting a learning environment, namely:

1 the people, such as the team leader, team members, student and mentors;
2 learning opportunities and experiences provided through clinical activities;
3 staff commitment to teaching (supervision) and learning (CPD); and
4 material resources.

Both above authors expressly avoid too much focus on learning environments as places where students merely achieve their course objectives, which policy definitions such as that of the NMC (2008b) do.

Earlier studies on clinical learning environments explored how effectively and deficiently learning occurs in practice settings. It formed the focus of research study by various authors, some of the earliest being by Fretwell (1980) and Orton (1981). The recommendations from these studies have been implemented fairly widely. From her study of practice settings as learning environments, Fretwell (1980) deduced that the key components of the 'ideal learning environment' are anti-hierarchy, teamwork, negotiation, communication and availability of trained nurses; and the practice setting sister's leadership in teaching is crucial in maintaining a learning ethos on the area.

Orton's (1981) study concluded with the identification of the characteristics of wards that are high student-oriented and those that were low student-orientated. In the former, all individuals in the practice setting including students and patients were manifestly valued, and staff showed willingness to teach. In the latter however, there was a lack of open-mindedness, lack of respect for individuals, and the atmosphere was not relaxed which made students anxious about asking questions. The responses in these earlier studies could be categorised as key factors that promote learning in the practice setting, and those that hinder, a number of which are identified in Box 11.1.

Box 11.1: Factors that promote learning and those that hinder learning in the practice setting

Factors that promote learning

- Teacher's knowledge
- Adequate time to teach
- Explanation of procedures
- Practical demonstration of skills
- Students feel they can take their time to practise the skills
- A learning ethos
- Teaching on a one-to-one basis
- Adequate staffing levels
- Adequate planning and preparation
- Reinforcing learning resources and information
- Approachable staff

Factors that hinder learning

- Interruptions
- Busy ward area
- Lack of time
- Staff, patient and learners' attitudes
- Availability of relevant medical equipments such as hoists
- Not enough information communicated
- Learner–staff ratio too high
- Inadequate staffing levels
- Student not interested
- Disorganised programme of teaching
- Poor leadership

Rotem and Hart's (1995) findings are also consistent with the above research findings in that some practice settings and institutions are found to be more conducive to learning than others. Later studies focused on exploring the extent to which particular practice settings were suitable for students' practice placements, and therefore on educational auditing (also known as the learning environment profile). For example, Orton et al. (1993), identified various components or criteria under orientation to the placement, theory and practice, supernumerary status, staff attitudes and behaviour, the mentor and progressive assessment. The ENB/DH (2001) *Placements in Focus* guidance identified such criteria under four key headings, namely: providing practice placements, practice learning environment, student support and assessment of practice. Under practice learning environment, the criteria include, for instance:

- The practice area should have a stated philosophy of care which is reflected in practice and in the curriculum aims.
- Care provision should be founded on relevant research-based and evidence-based findings where available.
- Students should gain, where possible, experience as part of a multiprofessional team.

- A learning resources area with relevant materials should be available for learning activities in the practice environment.
- Student feedback should be actively sought.

 Action point 11.5 – The 'learning environment profile' of your practice setting

Consider the learning ethos in your practice setting, and complete a SWOT analysis of the setting as a learning environment using the proforma presented below.

Alternatively, or additionally, Locate your practice setting's copy of the 'learning environment profile' (education audit) document to complete this action point.

STRENGTHS	WEAKNESSES
THREATS	OPPORTUNITIES

Other than in hospital wards, based on the first-hand experience of community nurses, Gopee et al. (2004) identify other specific requirements for enhancing primary care settings as effective clinical learning environments. This includes mentor–mentee matching in accordance with the seniority of the practitioner and the student's particular learning needs, ensuring that particular student practice outcomes are achievable within particular primary care settings, together with access to clinical supervision for all qualified staff.

Learning environment profiles also invite healthcare practitioners to identify formal and informal learning opportunities in each practice setting. These include teaching during care delivery or clinical interventions, that is, WBL, talks by medical device representatives, lectures or seminars presented by doctors, and opportunistic learning such as when a patient with a new condition is admitted. Such learning opportunities need to be recognised and nurtured by the DCM to ensure that the learning ethos endures.

For some decades, the responsibility for ensuring that clinical learning environments are suitable as practice placement areas has been that of the particular higher education institution offering the pre- and post-registration courses, but from 2006 this is the responsibility of healthcare trusts (NMC, 2008b).

The factors that are important for the creation of a positive learning environment include friendly staff, positive attitude and allocated time for teaching. Good communication is of course paramount, as is the learner feeling that they are part of the team. Staff reflecting up-to-date knowledge of the latest research in their specialism generally portray a positive impression. The availability and accessibility of research literature in the working environment may be kept in the learning resources section or in a resource room and also creates a positive image.

Furthermore, you might have noted that staff showing genuine interest in students' individual learning needs, and their stage of knowledge and competence development also creates positive impressions. The enthusiasm of all those who teach in practice settings and practice educators' input generate impetus for learning, and constructive criticism in an appropriate environment which is usually appreciated by students. A culture in which clinical staff are open to new ideas and share new learning from courses also present healthy perspectives, as is good staff morale.

From the DCM's perspective, learning in the practice setting needs to be approached from a management perspective including evaluation, analysis, introducing changes and so on.

 Action point 11.6 – Analysis of a practice setting as a learning environment

Following on from Action point 11.2, this exercise involves identifying actions that can be taken in respect of reviewing the effectiveness of your practice setting as a learning environment and identifying objectives and strategies for ensuring that they are effective. Consequently, consider your thoughts on the actions that you can take as a DCM to enhance your practice setting as a learning environment.

More recent studies on practice settings as learning environments focus on specific aspects of learning in practice settings. Lewin (2007) reports on a study evaluating five key components of effective learning environments comprising of the grade of staff students worked with most, how often practical procedures were demonstrated to them, and undertaken with them, how much of the time they were personally supervised and how often they worked with mentors who assessed them. This study, which is a replication of another study that was undertaken 25 years earlier, revealed a 20 per cent improvement in the five component areas.

Andrews et al. (2006) explored students' experiences during clinical placements, and concluded that commitment, collective vision, coordination and effective communication are crucially important requirements for successful practice placement experiences. Another perspective is provided by Henderson et al. (2006) who found that the psycho-social support available to students during clinical placements plays a very significant role.

The components identified specifically for ascertaining the extent to which practice settings are learning environments comprise frameworks or models of clinical learning environments. Various such frameworks extracted from research and in policy documents are available. Lewin's (2007) five-component framework of learning environments is one, Orton et al.'s (1993) is another, those identified by the ENB/DH (2001) is yet another, as are those in the trust-university education audit (or learning environment profile) documents.

Work-based learning and reflective learning

It has long been recognised that healthcare practitioners develop their competence through learning-by-doing in work settings, which includes learning clinical skills that might be assessed and signed by the mentor, and also accredited. Thus the concept and role of work-based learning (or practice-based learning) has been evolving and increasingly recognised in healthcare professions. Such learning is recognised in module details of healthcare profession courses, and therefore also commands a specific number of academic credit points.

Guile and Young (1996) amongst others suggest that WBL as a concept is innovative in that it places firm emphasis on the importance of the workplace as a site of learning, and Flanagan et al. (2000) note that it is a team-based, structured and learner-managed approach to maximising opportunities for learning and professional development in the workplace.

Some of the issues related to WBL include (Guile and Young, 1996) the limitations of the concept competence, which can reflect behaviourist assumptions and reductionist descriptions of work performance (i.e. simply as tasks), and therefore overlook theoretical knowledge; and comparability and equivalence between academic and work-based learning.

Furthermore, the Open University (2006) notes that work-based learning is a rather vague term in that it has been variously interpreted as learning that takes place in the workplace, learning that is based on the workplace and learning for the workplace. 'Workplace' sometimes refers to a specific place of work, at other times to signify that learning should have general benefits for practice. There is very little research on the benefits of any of these three forms. Nonetheless, WBL is supported by professional regulatory bodies, such as the NMC (2008b), and by the DH's *NHS KSF* (2004a) framework as it enhances the likelihood of 'fitness for practise' on qualifying, and supports lifelong learning.

The practice setting as a learning organisation

It was argued in Chapter 8 that social capital thrives in settings that reflect the features of a learning organisation. The work environment in which healthcare practitioners deliver care seems to have considerable effect on their learning.

The learning organisation (or the learning company) as a concept goes beyond the notion of the clinical environment in that it signifies support for learning from higher level structures such as the management team of an acute NHS trust. A learning organisation therefore implies that a learning attitude prevails in the management structure and strategies of the organisation itself.

Impinging on how much the clinical area as an organisation functions as a learning organisation is organisational culture, which in turn has an effect on staff morale, and on how conflict is resolved. Watkins and Marsick (1992:118) note that a learning organisation is characterised by 'total employee involvement in a process of collaboratively initiated, collaboratively conducted, collectively accountable change of direction towards shared values and principles'. Bahn (2001:115) discusses this in the context of social learning theory, and notes that the social environment has considerable impact on the 'collaborative approach to learning through the use of peers and expert practitioners as role models'. This is also related to the concept 'informal organisation' which refers to non-formal structures that constitute a powerful force in shaping culture in organisations.

Davies (1990) suggests that such mediums foster activities to help creativity. Increasing access to the Internet in the clinical area for literature searching and locating critically reviewed material can itself constitute informal peer-education. Internet facilities may be available in the practice setting's resource room or the staff room for informal social learning, or in the post-graduate department. The role of peer review and peer-assessment is explored quite comprehensively in Chapter 8.

The notion of the practice setting being a learning organisation has not been as widely researched and documented as the 'clinical learning environment'. However, as is obvious from the foregoing discussion on learning in practice settings, and concepts discussed in Chapter 8, that learning needs to be a fundamental underlying component of all activities in practice settings. It must not be a superficial add-on activity, but an intrinsic facet that ultimately ensures more informed patient care. It should be a feature of organisational culture in healthcare organisations. Staff development strategies should already be built into the organisational business plans, and are also evident in various DH policies and guidelines (e.g. DH, 1998, 2000d, 2001c). It is therefore well ingrained into the psycho-social ethos, and organisational culture of healthcare Trusts.

The learning culture in practice settings

According to the dictionary (Brown, 2002), culture refers to the distinctive customs, achievements, products and outlook of a group, their way of life. Organisational culture is defined by Huczynski and Buchanan (2007:623) as 'the collection of relatively uniform and enduring values, beliefs, customs, traditions, and practices that are shared by an organisation's members, learned by new recruits, and transmitted from one generation of employees to the next'. This definition clearly suggests recognising local attitudes that are ingrained and enduring, but focuses on the achievement of both the organisation's and its employees' goals for the organisation.

Mullins (2007) notes that culture is created and sustained through particular patterns of communication, values and beliefs that determine particular patterns of behaviour, and unconsciously held basic assumptions that determine group members' perceptions and feelings about modes of interactions within the organisation, along with the dynamics of the informal organisation. Four types of organisational culture are identified by Handy (1993), ranging from power culture, role, task or person cultures.

Power culture Refers to a setting in which power is vested generally in one individual, or in a small group of individuals, who control all activities of the organisation.

Role culture Refers to an organisational culture in which each employee's role and functions are clearly demarcated, and wherein work is allocated on the basis of their ability to do the task.

Task culture Refers to a product oriented culture, wherein the whole focus is on getting the job done, which involves appointing individuals with the right skills, and letting them get on with the job.

Person culture Refers to an organisation that heeds the basic needs of each individual employee.

 Action point 11.7 – Organisational culture

Which of these types of organisational culture prevail in your practice setting? How far does the identified culture(s) support a lasting learning ethos in your workplace?

Kane-Urrabazo (2006) notes that regardless of the four types of culture, there are also three critical components of organisational culture namely: (1) trustworthiness and trust, (2) empowerment and delegation, (3) consistency and mentorship, all of which influence employees' job satisfaction, and consequently organisational effectiveness. She suggests that managers should install support systems and mechanisms that enable employees' growth and development.

It is important, however, to distinguish between organisational culture and organisational climate, two concepts that are at times used interchangeably. Culture is something that endures over very long periods of time, while climate refers to more transient and changeable conditions. Increasingly this includes effective inter-professional learning.

Managing continuing learning

Having examined how practice settings can be effective learning environments and learning organisations, and then the mechanisms for developing and educating the workforce on a lifelong spectrum; this section explores how policy-directed learning can be achieved and how this interfaces with professional regulation.

The *Investors in People* award

A learning culture in the practice setting that is supported by an appropriately devised operational strategy directly impacts on the extent of formal and informal learning and also on achievement of the *Investors in People* (IIP) award. The 'Investors in People Standard' (Investors in People UK, 2004) comprises three key principles, ten indicators and a number of 'evidence requirements' against which organisations (or smaller units or departments) are assessed for the IIP award. The key principles are:

1 developing strategies to improve the performance of the organisation;
2 taking action to improve the performance of the organisation; and
3 evaluating the impact on the performance of the organisation.

These principles and indicators focus on people management, such as employee involvement and empowerment, reward and recognition. It involves the capability of leaders and managers being more closely measured. The IIP assessor looks to see how plans for professional education and CPD figure in the organisation's strategic plans, and how the impact of learning and development upon performance is measured and evaluated.

Mandatory learning and regulating healthcare practitioners

Another dimension of managing learning is mandatory learning. This notion, as a mechanism for CPD, is well known in nursing and midwifery circles in the form of post-registration education and practice (known as PREP) which has been in force for a number of years. It entails the registrant self-declaring to the NMC that they have updated their knowledge and competence, and therefore are allowed to remain on the register and to practise in that capacity; furthermore, registrants are expected to be lifelong learners (e.g. DH, 2001c). Doctors are expected to undertake similar activities (e.g. GMC, 2006), as are allied health professionals (e.g. HPC, 2006) and others (e.g. DH, 2004b).

The requirement for continuing education, revalidation and professional regulation of healthcare registrants has been evolving over time. The NMC was established in 2002, replacing the UKCC, to self-regulate the nursing and midwifery professions. The other eight regulatory bodies for healthcare practitioners in the United Kingdom are (HPC, 2006):

1 General Chiropractic Council
2 General Dental Council
3 General Medical Council
4 General Optical Council
5 General Osteopathic Council
6 Health Professions Council
7 Royal Pharmaceutical Society of Great Britain
8 Pharmaceutical Society of Northern Ireland.

Furthermore, social care professionals are regulated by the General Social Care Council. The Council for Healthcare Regulatory Excellence was established in 2003 to promote consistency across the nine regulatory bodies. However, there have been strong recommendations for more central regulation of healthcare professions. The DCM needs to be aware of this as the new proposed rules will directly impact on their day-to-day roles.

The government white paper *Trust, Assurance and Safety – The Regulation of Health Professionals in the 21st Century* (DH, 2007c) comprises a major development that outlines how healthcare professions will be regulated next. It sets out a programme of reform that is based on consultation of two reviews of professional regulation, one by the Chief Medical Officer published in July 2006 entitled *Good Doctors, Safer Patients* and another known as the Foster Report by the DH entitled *The Regulation of the Non-Medical Healthcare Professions*, and other contemporary reports of incompetence on the part of some healthcare practitioners. It is complemented by the government's response to the Shipman Inquiry and similar reports.

However, healthcare regulatory bodies such as the NMC, HPC and GMC in conjunction with health unions such as UNISON resisted central regulation until recently (Kendall-Raynor, 2006). This was because of a fear that professional regulation led by government departments might not be as insightful regarding the whys and hows of clinical interventions and might impose inappropriate penalties on suspected poor performance, for instance, than professional regulators might do. Professional development imposed by central regulators could be undertaken less wholeheartedly than if they were imposed by professional self-regulators.

The white paper in essence however proposes that the responsibility for ensuring that nurses are up to date should be transferred from the NMC to healthcare employers, thus replacing PREP by another system linked to the *NHS KSF*.

Managing funding for learning

It is up to the registrant to ensure they are up to date and competent in their clinical activities. However, it is one of the roles of the DCM to ascertain the skill needs of the practice setting and match them with the CPD interests of individual employees. The issues discussed in the preceding sections relates to the point that healthcare dynamics can affect learning in practice settings and indicate that learning and teaching in practice settings need to be managed and resourced.

The *NHS KSF* (DH, 2004a), for instance, clearly identifies the functions of groups of members of staff, and the professional development requirements and aspirations of each employee through IDPR. These can be documented in personal development plans, which are usually based on IDPRs.

Formal education programmes for healthcare practitioners are generally funded by local SHAs through 'funding' which identifies yearly budgets for this for each NHS trust. Created by the government in 2002 to manage the local NHS on behalf of the Secretary of State, there were originally 28 SHAs in England, and the number was reduced to ten in 2006 with the rationale that fewer and therefore more strategic organisations will deliver stronger commissioning functions, leading to improved services for patients and better value for money for the taxpayer. SHAs' roles were identified in Chapter 7. One of the key functions of SHA's is to identify funding for initial professional educational preparation and for post-registration professional development.

Guidelines for managing learning in the practice setting

The criteria contained within the 'learning environment profile' (educational audit) form, as well as those required for achieving the IIP award, together with other various policy documents constitute guidelines for good practice for sustaining a learning ethos in the practice setting.

Chapter summary

This chapter has focused on the DCM's role in ensuring that continuing learning occurs in the practice setting. This entailed examining:

- the route the newly qualified registrant, takes in progressing from being a healthcare practitioner to becoming a DCM, which includes being a preceptee to learning to become a manager, which in turn includes supervising learning;
- how to create, maintain and develop a learning ethos in practice settings, which includes the registrant's professionalism and CPD, and developing learning opportunities for healthcare practitioners and learners, the practice setting as a learning environment, work-based or practice-based learning and reflective learning, practice settings as learning organisations and a learning culture in practice settings; and
- how to achieve the IIP award, mandatory continuing learning and professional regulation by various agencies, and managing learning in practice settings, as well as guidelines for sustaining the learning ethos in practice settings.

Glossary

Care	Is used as a generic term that also represents therapy and treatment
Clinical support worker	Healthcare staff who are not registered with a professional regulatory body. Also known as healthcare assistant, healthcare support worker
Duty clinical manager	Is the term used throughout the book to refer to a healthcare professional that has management responsibility for a group of patients, a team of staff or a practice setting. The responsibility may be for the duration of a span of duty, for example, managing the practice setting, or may be more permanent in nature, for example, managing a team of staff or a group of patients. The term is used as a way of differentiating between the role and responsibilities of the identified figurehead or appointed manager of the practice setting
Efficiency	The achievement of expected objectives at minimum financial costs, in the minimum amount of time, but of the required standard
Effectiveness	The achievement of expected patient outcomes
Healthcare organisation	Acute NHS trusts, Primary Care Trusts (PCT), Teaching PCTs, GP practices, Nursing Homes, etc.
Healthcare practitioner/ healthcare professional	Refers to an individual healthcare professional registered with their appropriate regulatory body e.g. nurse, physiotherapist
Manpower equivalents (MPE)	MPE relates to the total number of staff hours expressed as a percentage of full-time positions
Patient	Used a generic term to refer to 'users' of health and social care in the widest sense and therefore also represents service users and clients
Practice setting	Relates to the locations where healthcare practitioners deliver care, to include wards, clinics, GP surgeries and the patients own home etc.
Registrant	Used interchangeably with 'healthcare practitioner' and 'healthcare professional', registrant refers to

qualified nurses, doctors, allied health professionals and health scientists, etc. who are registered with their respective professional bodies

Skill mix

A term that refers to the numbers and ratio, capability and experience of qualified and unqualified staff, which in the case of nursing are required to meet the nursing component of healthcare

Span of duty

Relates to the duration of time that the practitioner is on duty e.g. the duration of their shift

References

Adair J (2005) *Effective Leadership Development*. London: Chartered Institute of Personnel and Development.

Alexander C (1997) 'Influencing decision making'. *Nursing Standard*, 11 (38): 39–44.

Almio-Metcalf B (1996) 'Leaders or managers'. *Nursing Management*, 3 (1): 22–24.

American Nurses Association (ANA) and National Council of State Boards of Nursing (NCSBN) (2005) *Joint Statement on Delegation*. Available from: nursingworld.org/search/vfp_search.cfm (accessed 12 July 2007).

Andrews G J, Brodie D A, Andrews J P, Hillan E, Thomas B G, Wong J and Rixon L (2006) 'Professional roles and communications in clinical placements: a qualitative study of nursing students' perceptions and some models for practice'. *International Journal of Nursing Studies*, 43 (7): 861–874.

Anonymous (1998) 'Great expectations'. *Nursing Times*, 94 (30): 66–67.

Armstrong M (2006) *A Handbook of Human Resource Management Practice* (10th edn). London: Kogan Page. Also available from: www.answers.com/topic/human-resource-management?cat=biz-fin (accessed 23 July 2007).

Atwal A and Caldwell K (2006) 'Nurses' perceptions of multidisciplinary team work in acute health-care'. *International Journal of Nursing Practice*, 12 (6): 359–365.

Bahn D (2001) 'Social learning theory: its application in the context of nurse education'. *Nurse Education Today*, 21 (2): 110–117.

Bain L (1996) 'Preceptorship: a review of literature'. *Journal of Advanced Nursing*, 24 (1): 104–107.

Ballard J (1994) 'District nurses – who's looking after them?' *Occupational Health Review*, 52 (Nov/Dec): 10–19.

Baron S, Field J and Schuller T (eds) (2000) *Social Capital: Critical Perspectives*. Oxford: Oxford University Press.

Barr H (2002) *Interprofessional Education Today, Yesterday and Tomorrow: A Review*. London: LTSN HS&P.

Bass B M (1990) *Bass and Stogdill's Handbook of Leadership: Theory, Research and Managerial Applications* (3rd edn). New York, Free Press.

Bass B M and Riggio R E (2006*) Transformational leadership*. London, Lawrence Erlbaum Associates.

Beckhard R and Harris R T (1987) *Organisational Transitions: Managing Complex Change*. (2nd edn). Massachusetts: Addison-Wesley.

Belbin RM (1993) Team Roles At Work Elsevier / Butterworth Heinemann. Chapter 3 p.22 and www.belbin.com

Benner P (2001) *From Novice to Expert: Excellence and Power in Clinical Nursing Practice*. London/California: Addison-Wesley.

Bennis W and Nanus B (1985) *Leaders: The Strategies for Taking Charge*. New York: Harper and Row.

Berne E (1975) *What Do You Say After You Say Hello?* London: Corgi Books.

Binnie A (1998) 'How to grow more leaders'. *Nursing Times*, 94 (28): 24–26.

Bishop V (1998) 'Clinical supervision: what's going on? Results of a questionnaire survey'. *Nursing Times*, 94 (18): 50–53.

Blake R R and McCanse A A (1991) *Leadership Dilemmas – Grid Solutions*. Houston: Gulf Publishing Company.

Bond M and Holland S (1998) *Skills in Clinical Supervision for Nurses: A Practical Guide for Supervisees, Clinical Supervisors and Managers*. Buckingham: Open University Press.

Borrill C S, West M A, Shapiro D and Rees A (2000) 'Team working and effectiveness in health care'. *British Journal of Health Care Management*, 6 (8): 534–535.

Boud D, Keogh R and Walker D (Eds) (1985) *Reflection: Turning Experience into Learning*. London: Kogan Page. [Reprinted 2002].

Bowles N and Young C (1999) 'An evaluative study of clinical supervision based on Proctor's three function interactive model'. *Journal of Advanced Nursing*, 30 (4): 958–964.

Brashers D E, Haas S M and Neidig J L (1999) 'The Patient Self-Advocacy Scale: measuring patient involvement in health care decision-making interactions'. *Health Communication*, 11(2): 97–121.

Brown L (editor-in-chief) (2002) *Shorter Oxford English Dictionary* (5th edn). Oxford: Oxford University Press.

Brown P (1998) 'Endangered species'. *The Times*, 29 October 1998, p. 2.

Bryans P and Cronin T P (1983) *Organization Theory*. London: Mitchell Beazley.

Bryar R M and Griffiths J M (eds) (2003) *Practice Development in Community Nursing*. London: Arnold.

Burnard P and Morrison P (2005) 'Nurses' perceptions of their interpersonal skills: a descriptive study using six category intervention analysis'. *Nurse Education Today*, 25 (8): 612–617.

Byrne M W and Keefe M R (2002) 'Building research competence in nursing through mentoring'. *Journal of Nursing Scholarship*, 34 (4): 391–396.

Cahill J (1996) 'Patient participation: a concept analysis'. *Journal of Advanced Nursing*, 24 (3): 561–571.

Cairns J (1998) 'Clinical supervision and the practice nurse'. *Journal of Community Nursing*, 12 (9): 20–24.

Caldwell K, Atwall A, Copp G, Brett-Richards M and Coleman K (2006) 'Preparing for practice: how well are practitioners prepared for teamwork'. *British Journal of Nursing*, 15 (22): 1250–1254.

Calpin-Davies F (2000) 'Nurse manager, change thyself'. *Nursing Management*, 6 (9): 16–20.

Campbell C, Wood R and Kelly M (1999) *Social Capital and Health*. London: Health Education Authority.

Canadian Health Services Research Foundation (CHSRF) (2006) *Teamwork in Healthcare: Promoting Effective Teamwork in Healthcare in Canada*. Ontario: CHSRF.

Carper B A (1978) 'Fundamental patterns of knowing in nursing'. *Advances in Nursing Science*, 1 (1): 13–23.

Carroll H (1997) 'Developing a protocol for clinical practice'. *British Journal of Renal Medicine*, (Autumn 1997): 25–27.

Carver N, Ashmore R and Clibbens N (2006) 'Group clinical supervision in pre-registration nurse training: the views of mental health nursing students'. *Nurse Education Today*, 27 (7): 768–776.

Castle A (2007) 'Lean thinking on the wards'. *Nursing Standard*, 22 (8): 16–18.

Centre for Policy on Ageing (2007) *Single Assessment Process – Moving Towards a Common Assessment Framework*. Available from: www.cpa.org.uk/sap/sap_home.html (accessed 2 March 2008).

Charns M P and Tewksbury L S (1993) *Collaborative Management in Health Care: Implementing the Integrating Organisation*. San Francisco: Jossey-Bass.

Chief Nursing Officer (CNO) (2002) *Implementing the NHS plan – Ten Key Roles for Nurses (PL CNO (2002)5)*. Available from: www.dh.gov.uk/en/Publicationsandstatistics/Lettersandcirculars/Professionalletters/Chiefnursingofficerletters/DH_4004780 (accessed 11 November 2007).

Clarke A, Hanson EJ and Ross H (2003) 'Seeing the person behind the patient: enhancing the care of older people using a biographical approach'. *Journal of Clinical Nursing,* 12 (5): 697–706.

Clegg A (2000) 'Leadership: improving the quality of patient care'. *Nursing Standard,* 14 (30): 43–45.

Clinical Governance Support Team (2007) *About CG – What Is Clinical Governance?* Available from: www.cgsupport.nhs.uk/About_CG/ (accessed 11 November 2007).

Collinson G (2000) 'Encouraging the growth of the nurse entrepreneur'. *Professional Nurse,* 15 (6): 365–367.

Cook M J (2001) 'The attributes of effective clinical nurse leaders'. *Nursing Standard,* 18 (35): 33–36.

Cook M J and Leathard H L (2004) 'Learning for clinical leadership'. *Journal of Nursing Management,* 12 (6): 436–444.

Covey S (1992) *Principle-Centred Leadership.* New York: Simon and Schuster Inc.

Cunningham G and Kitson A (2000) 'An evaluation of the RCN Clinical Leadership Development Programme'. *Nursing Standard,* (part 1) 15 (12): 34–37 and (part 2) 15 (13): 34–40.

Curtis E and Nicholl H (2004) 'Delegation: a key function of nursing'. *Nursing Management,* 11 (4): 26–31.

Darley M (1995) 'Clinical supervision: the view from the top'. *Nursing Management,* 2 (3): 14–15.

Davies C (1990) *The Collapse of the Conventional Career. The Future of Work and Its Relevance for Post-Registration Education in Nursing, Midwifery and Health Visiting.* English Nursing Board (ENB) Project Paper 3. London: ENB.

Dearlove D (1997) 'No substitute for bright ideas'. *The Times,* 3 July 1997, p. 5.

Department of Health (DH) (1991) *The Patient's Charter.* London: The Stationery Office.

Department of Health (DH) (1993) *Clinical Audit: Meeting and Improving Standards.* London: The Stationery Office.

Department of Health (DH) (1997) *The New NHS: Modern, Dependable.* London: The Stationery Office.

Department of Health (DH) (1999) *Making a Difference.* London: The Stationery Office.

Department of Heath (DH) (2000a) *The NHS Plan: A Plan for Investment, a Plan for Reform.* London: The Stationery Office.

Department of Health (DH) (2000b) *Improving Working Lives Standard.* London: The Stationery Office.

Department of Health (DH) (2000c) *A Health Service for All the Talents: Developing NHS Workforce.* London: The Stationery Office.

Department of Health (DH) (2000d) *An Organisation with a Memory: Report of an Expert Group on Learning from Adverse Events in the NHS Chaired by the Chief Medical Officer.* London: The Stationery Office. Available from: Www.dh.gov.uk/PublicationsAndStatistics/ (accessed 11 March 2007).

Department of Health (DH) (2001a) *Health and Social Care Act.* London: The Stationery Office.

Department of Health (DH) (2001b) *National Service Framework for Older People.* London: The Stationery Office.

Department of Health (DH) (2001c) *Expert Patient Programme.* London: The Stationery Office.

Department of Health (DH) (2001d) *Working Together – Learning Together. A Framework for Lifelong Learning for the NHS.* London: The Stationery Office.

Department of Health (DH) (2002) *Liberating the Talents: Helping Primary Care Trusts and Nurses to Deliver the NHS Plan.* Available from: www.doh.gov.uk/cno/liberatingtalents.htm (accessed 11 November 2007).

Department of Health (DH) (2003) *The Essence of Care: Patient Focused Benchmarks for Clinical Governance*. London: The Stationery Office.

Department of Health (DH) (2004a) *NHS Knowledge and Skills Framework*. Available from: www. dh.gov.uk/en/Publicationsandstatistics/Publications/PublicationsPolicyAndGuidance/ DH_4090843 (accessed 15 July 2007).

Department of Health (DH) (2004b) *The NHS Improvement Plan: Putting People at the Heart of Public Services*. London: The Stationery Office.

Department of Health (DH) (2004c) *Agenda for Change*. London: The Stationery Office.

Department of Health (DH) (2004d) *Patient and Public Involvement in Health: A Summary of the Results of the Health in Partnership Research Programme*. London: The Stationery Office.

Department of Health (DH) (2004e) *Choosing Health: Making Healthy Choices Easier*. London: The Stationery Office.

Department of Health (DH) (2005a) *National Service Frameworks*. Available from: www.dh.gov. uk/PolicyAndGuidance/HealthAndSocialCareTopics/ (accessed 18 November 2007).

Department of Health (DH) (2005b) *Creating a Patient-led NHS: Delivering the NHS Improvement Plan*. London: The Stationery Office.

Department of Health (DH) (2006a) *Our Health, Our Care, Our Say: A New Direction for Community Services*. London: The Stationery Office.

Department of Health (DH) (2006b) *Standards for Better Health*. Available from: www.dh. gov.uk/ (accessed 20 September 2007).

Department of Health (DH) (2006c) *Modernising Nursing Careers: Setting the Direction*. London: The Stationery Office.

Department of Health (DH) (2006d) *From Values to Action: The Chief Nursing Officer's Review of Mental Health Nursing*. Available from: www.dh.gov.uk/en/Publicationsandstatistics/ Publications/PublicationsPolicyAndGuidance/DH_4133839 <http://www.dh.gov.uk/en/ Publicationsandstatistics/Publications/PublicationsPolicyAndGuidance/DH_4133839> (accessed 28 July 2008).

Department of Health (DH) (2006e) *The Chief Medical Officer on the State of Public Health Annual Report 2005*. London: The Stationery Office.

Department of Health (DH) (2006f) *Your Health, Your Care, Your Say*. Available from: www. dh.gov.uk/ (accessed 20 September 2007).

Department of Health (DH) (2007a) *Shaping Healthcare for the Next Decade (led by Lord Darzi)*. Available from: www.gnn.gov.uk/ (accessed 8 July 2007).

Department of Health (DH) (2007b) *Good Practice in Learning Disability Nursing*. Available from: www.dh.gov.uk/en/Publicationsandstatistics/Publications/PublicationsPolicy And Guidance/DH_081328 (accessed 30 June 2008).

Department of Health (DH) (2007c) *Trust, Assurance and Safety – The Regulation of Health Professionals in the 21st Century* White Paper. Available from: www.dh.gov.uk/ PublicationsAndStatistics/ (accessed 11 March 2007).

Department of Health (DH) (2007d) *NHS Foundation Trusts*. Available from: www.dh. gov.uk/ en/Policyandguidance/Organisationpolicy/Secondarycare/NHSfoundationtrust/index.htm (accessed 27 August 2007).

Department of Health (DH) (2007e) *Essence of Care: Benchmarks for the Care Environment*. Available from: www.dh.gov.uk/en/Publicationsandstatistics/Publications/ PublicationsPolicyAnd Guidance /DH_080058 (accessed 11 March 08).

Department of Health (DH) (2007f) *Making Experiences Count: A New Approach to Responding to Complaints*. London: The Stationery Office.

Department of Health (DH) (2007g) *How DH Works: Managing the System*. Available from: www.dh.gov.uk/en/Aboutus/HowDHworks/DH_074634 (accessed 16 September 2007).

Department of Health (DH) (2007h) *Payment by Results*. Available from: www.dh.gov.uk/en/Policyandguidance/Organisationpolicy/Financeandplanning/NHSFinancialReforms/index.htm (accessed: 29 October 2007).

Department of Health (DH) (2008a) *High Quality Care For All – NHS Next Stage Review Final Report*. Available from: www.dh.gov.uk/en/Publications andstatistics/Publications/PublicationsPolicyAndGuidance/DH_085825 (accessed 10 July 2008).

Department of Health (DH) (2008b) *A Consultation on the NHS Constitution*. Available from: http://www.dh.gov.uk/en/Consultations/Liveconsultations/DH_085812 (accessed 15 July 2008).

Dickson R (1996) 'Dissemination and implementation: the wider picture'. *Nurse Researcher*, 4 (1): 5–14.

Donabedian A (1988) 'The quality of care. How can it be assessed?' *American Journal of Public Health*, 260 (12): 1743.

Drennan V (2007) Nurse, Midwife and Health Visitor Entrepreneurship in the UK. Paper Presented at The 2007 International Nursing Research Conference, Dundee.

Driscoll J (2000) *Practising Clinical Supervision. A Reflective Approach*. London: Bailliere Tindall.

Driscoll J and Cooper R (2005) 'Coaching for clinicians'. *Nursing Management*, 12 (1): 18–23.

Drucker P F (1979) *Management*. London: Pan Books.

Duff L (1998) 'The RCN strategy on clinical guidelines'. *Nursing Standard*, 13 (8): 33–34.

Dukes J and Stewart R (1993) 'Be prepared'. *Health Services Journal*, 103 (5337): 24–25.

Dunn S V and Hansford B (1997) 'Undergraduate nursing students' perceptions of their clinical learning environment'. *Journal of Advanced Nursing*, 25 (6): 1299–1306.

Duxbury J and Whittington R (2005) 'Causes and management of patient aggression and violence: staff and patient perspectives'. *Journal of Advanced Nursing*, 50 (5): 469–478.

Ellis J (1995) 'Using benchmarking to improve practice'. *Nursing Standard*, 9 (35): 25–28.

Ellis R B, Gates B and Kenworthy N (2003) *Interpersonal Communication in Nursing*. Edinburgh: Churchill Livingstone.

English National Board/Department of Health (2001) *Placements in Focus*. London: ENB/DH.

Evans L (2002) 'An exploration of district nurses' perception of occupational stress'. *British Journal of Nursing*, 11 (8): 576–585.

Faugier J and Woolnough H (2003) 'Lessons from LEO'. *Nursing Management*, 10 (2): 22–25.

Fayol, H. (1949) *General and Industrial Management*. (Translated from the French edition (Dunod) by Constance Storrs). Essex: Pitman/Pearson Education. Available from: www.hrmguide.co.uk/history/classical_organization_theory_modified.htm (accessed 7 March 2008).

Fields H (1994) 'Coaching and mentoring'. *Nursing Standard*, 8 (30): 105–111.

Field J (1999) 'Participation under the magnifying glass'. *Adults Learning* (November 1999), 11 (3): 10–13.

Filley A C (1975) *Interpersonal Conflict Resolution*. Glenview, Illinois: Scott & Foresman.

Finlayson B, Dixon J, Meadows S and Blair G (2002) 'Mind the gap: the policy response to the NHS nursing shortage'. *British Medical Journal*, 325 (7363): 541–544.

Flanagan J, Baldwin S and Clarke D (2000) 'Work-based learning as a means of developing and assessing nursing competence'. *Journal of Clinical Nursing*, 9 (3): 360–368.

Florin J, Ehrenberg A and Ehnfors M (2005) 'Patients' and nurses' perceptions of nursing problems in an acute setting'. *Journal of Advanced Nursing*, 51 (2):140–149.

Freeth D, Hammick M, Koppel I, Reeves S and Barr H (2002) *A Critical Review of Evaluations of Interprofessional Education. Learning and teaching Support Network*. Available from: www.health.ltsn.ac.uk/publications/occasionalpaper/occasionalpaper02.pdf (accessed 11 November 2007).

Fretwell, J E (1980) 'An inquiry into the ward learning environment'. *Nursing Times,* 26 June 1980, pp. 69–75.

Garbett R, Hardy S, Manley K, Titchen A and McCormack B (2007) 'Developing a qualitative approach to 360-degree feedback to aid understanding and development of clinical expertise'. *Journal of Nursing Management,* 15 (3): 342–347.

Garbett R and McCormack B (2002) 'A concept analysis of practice development'. *NTResearch,* 7 (2): 87–100.

General Medical Council (GMC) (2004) *Continuing Professional Development.* London: GMC.

General Medical Council (GMC) (2006) *Read the GMC Statement in response to Trust, Assurance and Safety – The Regulation of Health Professionals.* White Paper. Available from: www.gmc-uk.org/about/white_paper/index.asp (accessed 8 March 2007).

General Medical Council (GMC) (2007) *Doctors under Investigation – Performance Assessments.* Available from: http://www.gmc-uk.org/ (accessed 8 March 2007).

Gibbon B, Watkins C, Barber D, Waters K, Davies S, Lightbody L and Leathley M (2002) 'Can staff attitudes to team working in stroke care be improved?' *Journal of Advanced Nursing,* 40 (1):105–111.

Goldsmith M, Stewart L and Ferguson L (2006) 'Peer learning partnership: innovative strategy to enhance skill acquisition in nursing students'. *Nurse Education Today,* 26 (2): 123–130.

Goleman D (2000) 'Leadership that gets results'. *Harvard Business Review,* (March–April 2000) 78 (2): 78–90.

Gopee N (2000) 'Self-assessment and the concept of the lifelong learning nurse'. *British Journal of Nursing,* 9 (11): 724–729.

Gopee N (2001) 'Lifelong learning in nursing – perceptions and realities'. *Nurse Education Today,* 21 (8), 607–615.

Gopee N (2008) *Mentoring and Supervision in Healthcare.* London: Sage Publications.

Gopee N, Tyrrell A, Raven S, Thomas K and Hari T (2004) 'Effective clinical learning in primary care settings'. *Nursing Standard,* 18 (37): 33–37.

Gould D, Kelly D and Gouldstone L (2001) 'Preparing nurse managers to mentor students'. *Nursing Standard,* 16 (11): 39–42.

Gratton L (2000) *Living Strategy: Putting People at the Heart of Corporate Purpose.* London: Financial Times/Prentice Hall.

Gray J A M (2001) *Evidence-Based Healthcare. How to Make Policy and Management Decisions* (2nd edn). Edinburgh: Churchill Livingstone.

Greenleaf R K (1991) *The Servant as Leader.* Indianapolis: The Robert K Greenleaf Center.

Guile D and Young M (1996) 'Further professional development and further education teachers: setting a new agenda for work-based learning'. In Woodward I (1996) *Continuing Professional Development: Issues in Design and Delivery.* London: Cassell.

Gullick J, Shepherd B and Ronald T (2004) 'The effect of an organisational model on the standard of care'. *Nursing Times,* 100 (10): 36–39.

Hamm R M (1988) 'Clinical intuition and clinical analysis: expertise and the cognitive continuum'. In Dowie J and Elstein A (eds) (1988) *Professional Judgement: A Reader in Clinical Decision Making.* Milton Keynes: Open University Press.

Handy C (1984) *The Future of Work: A Guide to a Changing Society.* Oxford: Blackwell Publications.

Handy C (1993) *Understanding Organizations* (4th edn). Harmondsworth: Penguin Books Ltd.

Hawkins P and Shohet R (2006) *Supervision in the Helping Professions* (3rd edn). Berkshire: Open University Press.

Hayward J (1975) *Information – A Prescription against Pain.* London: RCN.

Health and Safety Executive (HSE) (1998) *Provision and Use of Work Equipment Regulations.* Available from: www.hse.gov.uk/pubns/indg291.pdf (accessed 26 June 2007).

Healthcare Commission (2005) *Acute Hospital Portfolio: Ward Staffing, Commission for Healthcare, Audit and Inspection*. London: Healthcare Commission.

Healthcare Commission (2006) *National Survey of NHS Staff 2005*. London: CHAI.

Healthcare Commission (2007) *Inpatients: The Views of Hospital Inpatients in England*. London: Healthcare Commission.

Health Professions Council (HPC) (2006) *Who Regulates Health and Social Care Professionals?* Available from: www.gdc-uk.org/ (accessed 2 April 2007).

Hellriegel D, Jackson S E and Slocum J W (2002) *Management: A Competency-based Approach* (9th edn). Cincinatti: South Western.

Henderson A, Twentyman M, Heel A and Lloyd B (2006) 'Students' perception of the psychosocial clinical learning environment: an evaluation of placement models'. *Nurse Education Today*, 26 (7): 564–571.

Heron J (1989) *Six Category Intervention Analysis. Human Potential Research Project* (2nd edn). Guildford: University of Surrey.

Herzberg F (1974) *Work and the Nature of Man*. London: Staples Press.

HM Treasury (2002) *Securing Our Future Health: Taking a Long-Term View*. The Wanless Report. Available from: http://www.hm-treasury.gov.uk/Consultations_and_ Legislation/ wanless/consult_ wanless_ final.cfm (accessed 9 May 2005).

HM Treasury (2007) *Budget 2007 – Summary Leaflet*. London: HM Teasury.

Hoeman S P (2002) *Rehabilitation Nursing: Process, Application and Outcomes*. St Louis (Missouri): Mosby.

Hollingsworth M J (1999) 'Purpose and values'. *The British Journal of Administrative Management*, January/February 1999, pp. 22–23.

Hollis V (1991) 'Self-directed learning as a post-basic educational continuum'. *British Journal of Occupational Therapy*, 54 (2): 45–48.

Howatson-Jones I L (2004) 'The servant leader'. *Nursing Management*, 11 (3): 20–24.

Huczynski A A and Buchanan D A (2007) *Organisational Behaviour* (6th edn). London: Prentice Hall/Financial Times.

Hunt J (1997) 'Towards evidence-based practice'. *Nursing Management*, 4 (2): 14–17.

Hurst K (2006) Nursing by numbers. *Nursing Standard*, 21 (7): 22-25.

Hyrkas K, Appelqvist-schmidlechner K and Kivimaki K (2005) 'First-line managers' views of the long-term effects of clinical supervision: how does clinical supervision support and develop leadership in health care?' *Journal of Nursing Management*, 13 (3): 209–220.

Institute for Healthcare Improvement (IHI) (2006) *She's Got a Ticket To … Go Home*. Available from: www.ihi.org/IHI/Topics/MedicalSurgicalCare/MedicalSurgicalCareGeneral/ ImprovementStories/ShesGotaTicketToGoHome.htm (accessed 27 August 2007).

Institute for Healthcare Improvement (IHI) (2007) *How to Improve – The Plan-Do-Study-Act (PDSA) Cycle* (Cambridge, USA). Available from: www.ihi.org/IHI/Topics/Improvement/ ImprovementMethods/HowToImprove/ (accessed 27 August 2007).

Institute for Medicine (1992) Guidelines for Clinical Practice: From Development to Use. Washington DC, National Academic Press.

Investors in People UK (IIP) (2004) *Unlock Your Organisation's Potential*. Available from: www. investorsinpeople.co.uk/ (accessed 2 April 2007).

Jarvis P and Gibson S (1997) *The Teacher Practitioner and Mentor* (2nd edn). Cheltenham: Stanley Thornes.

Johnson M and Webb C (1995) 'Rediscovering unpopular patients: the concept of social judgement'. *Journal of Advanced Nursing*, 21 (3): 466–475.

Jones A (2006) 'Clinical supervision: what do we know and what do we need to know? A review and commentary'. *Journal of Nursing Management*, 14 (8): 577–585.

Joseph Rowntree Foundation (2005) *Involving older People: What Standards Should We Expect*. York: Joseph Rowntree Foundation.

Kane-Urrabazo C (2006) 'Management's role in shaping organization culture'. *Journal of Nursing Management,* 14 (3): 188–194.

Katz D and Kahn R L (1952) 'Some recent findings in human relations research'. In Sullivan E J and Decker P J (2009) *Effective Leadership and Management in Nursing* (6th edn). London: Prentice Hall International.

Kendall-Raynor P (2006) 'Foster regulation proposals rejected by unions and NMC'. *Nursing Standard,* 21 (10): 5.

Kennedy I (2001) *Learning from Bristol: The Report of the Public inquiry into Children's Heart Surgery at the Bristol royal Infirmary 1984–1995.* London: The Stationery Office.

Kitwood T M (1997) *Dementia Reconsidered: The Person Comes First.* Buckingham: Open University Press.

Klakovich M D (1994) 'Connective leadership for the 21st century: a historical perspective and future directions'. *Advances in Nursing Science,* 16 (4): 42–54.

Kotter J P (1990) 'What leaders really do'. *Harvard Business Review,* May–June 1990, p. 103. In Mullins L J (2007) *Management and Organisational Behaviour* (8th edn). London: Financial Times/Prentice Hall.

Kouzes J M and Posner B Z (2007) *The Leadership Challenge* (4th edn). San Francisco: Jossey-Bass.

Kramer M (1974) *Reality Shock: Why Nurses Leave Nursing.* St Louis (Missouri): Mosby.

Lamb G S and Stempel J E (1994) 'Nurse case management from the client's view: growing as insider expert'. *Nursing Outlook,* 42 (1): 7–13.

Leathard A (2003) *Interprofessional Collaboration in Health and Social Care.* Sussex: Brunner-Routledge.

Leners D W, Wilson V W, Connor P and Fenton J (2006) 'Mentorship: increasing retention probabilities'. *Journal of Nursing Management,* 14 (8): 652–654.

Lewin D (2007) 'Clinical learning environments for student nurses: key indices from two studies compared over a 25 year period'. *Nurse Education in Practice,* 7 (4): 238–246.

Lewin K (1951) *Field Theory in Social Science.* London: Harper Row.

Liefer D (2005) 'My practice: Government policy changes allowed an entrepreneurial nurse to pave the way for nurse-led general practices'. *Nursing Standard,* 19 (22): 58.

Lipley N (2004) 'Two-year funding to train more leaders'. *Nursing Management,* 11 (6): 4.

Mackenzie J (ed.) (1998) *Ward Management in Practice.* Edinburgh: Churchill Livingstone.

Magnus O, Johansson P and Fridlund B (2004) 'Nursing care at night: an evaluation using the Night Nursing Care Instrument'. *Journal of Advanced Nursing,* 47 (1): 25–32.

Malby B and Manning S (1998) 'Promoting change through peer review'. *Nursing Management,* 5 (2): 24–25.

Malkin K F (1994) 'A standard for professional development: the use of self and peer review; learning contracts and reflection in clinical practice'. *Journal of Nursing Management,* 2: 143–148.

Manley K (1997) 'A conceptual framework for advanced practice: an action research project operationalizing and advanced practitioner/consultant nurse role'. *Journal of Clinical Nursing,* 6 (3): 179–190.

Marinker M, Blenkinsopp A, Bond C, Britten N and Feely M (1997) *From Compliance to Concordance: Achieving Shared Goals in Medicine Taking.* London: Royal Pharmaceutical Society of Great Britain.

Markham G (1998) 'Gender in leadership'. *Nursing Management,* 3 (1): 18–19.

Marquis B L and Huston C J (2006) *Leadership Roles and Management Functions in Nursing* (5th edn). Philadelphia: Lippincott Williams and Wilkins.

Marriner-Tomey A (2004) *Guide to Nursing Management and Leadership* (7th edn). St Louis (Missouri): Mosby.

Maslin-Prothero S (1997) 'A perspective on lifelong learning and its implications for nurses'. *Nurse Education Today,* 17 (6): 431–436.

Maslow A H (1987) *Motivation and Personality* (3rd edn). London: Harper and Row.

Maxwell R (1984) 'Quality assessment in health'. *British Medical Journal*, 288 (6428): 1470–1472.

McAllister M and Osborne Y (1997) 'Peer review – a strategy to enhance co-operative student learning'. *Nurse Educator*, 22 (1): 40–44.

McCaughan D (2002) 'What decisions do nurses make'. In Thompson C and Dowding D (eds) *Clinical Decision Making and Judgement in Nursing*. Edinburgh: Churchill Livingstone.

McClelland D (1975) *Power: The Inner Experience*. New York: Irvington.

McCormack B, Dewar B, Wright J, Garbett R, Harvey G and Ballantine K (2006) *A Realist Synthesis of Evidence Relating to Practice Development*. Available from: www.nhshealthquality. org (accessed 18 April 2007).

McGregor D (1987) *The Human Side of Enterprise*. Harmondsworth, Middlesex: Penguin.

McNichol E and Smith S (2001) 'Measure your leadership skills'. *Nursing Standard*, 15 (22): 77.

Meadows S, Levenson R and Baeza J (2000) *The Last Straw – Explaining the NHS Nursing Shortage*. London: King's Fund Centre.

Menzies I E (1960) 'A case study in the functioning of social systems as a defence against anxiety: a report of a study of nursing services of a general hospital'. *The Tavistock Institute of Human Relations*, 13 (2): 95–121.

Middleton S and Roberts A (ed.) (2000) *Integrated Care Pathways: A Practical Approach to Implementation*. Oxford: Butterworth Heinemann.

Mintzberg H (1990) *The Nature of Managerial Work*. London: Prentice Hall.

Morgan C (2005) 'Growing your own – a model for encouraging and nurturing aspiring leaders'. *Nursing Management*, 11 (9): 27–30.

Moroney N and Knowles C (2006) 'Innovation and teamwork: introducing multi-disciplinary team ward rounds'. *Nursing Management*, 13 (1): 28–31.

Morse J, Bottorff J, Anderson G, O'Brien B and Solberg S (1992) 'Beyond empathy: expanding expressions of caring'. *Journal of Advanced Nursing*, 17 (7): 809–821.

Morton Medical (2004) *Unistik 2 Single Use Needle Safe Capillary Blood Sampling Device*. Available from: www.mortonmedical.co.uk/Unistik_2 Capillary_Blood_Sampling_Device. htm (accessed 18 September 2007).

Mouton J S and Blake R R (1984) *Synergogy*. San Francisco: Jossey-Bass.

Mullins L J (2007) *Management and organisational behaviour* (8th edn). London: Financial Times/Prentice Hall.

Mumma C M and Nelson A (2002) 'Theory and practice models for rehabilitation nursing'. In Hoeman S P (2002) *Rehabilitation Nursing: Process, Application and Outcomes*. St Louis (Missouri): Mosby.

Murphy L (2005) 'Transformational leadership: a cascading chain reaction'. *Journal of Nursing Management*, 13 (2): 128–136.

National Health Service Litigation Authority (2007) *About the NHS Litigation Authority*. Available from: www.nhsla.com/home.htm (accessed 11 November 2007).

National Patient Safety Agency (2004) *Seven Steps to Patient Safety for Primary Care*. Available from: www.npsa.nhs.uk/health/resources/7steps (accessed 14 November 2007).

NHS Choice (2007) *About the NHS: Authorities and trusts*. Available from: www.nhs.uk/ aboutnhs/howtheNHSworks/authoritiesandtrusts/Pages/Authoritiesandtrusts.aspx (accessed 27 June 2007).

NHS Employers (2006a) *Stop Bullying: It's in Your Hands*. London: NHS Employers/Available from: www.nhsemployers.org/toolkit/search.cfm (accessed 5 March 2007).

NHS Employers (2006b) *Model Bullying and Harassment Policy*. London: NHS Employers/ Available from: www.nhsemployers.org/toolkit/search.cfm (accessed 5 March 2007).

NHS Executive (1996) *Clinical Guidelines*. Leeds: NHSE.

NHS Executive (1999) *Public Interest Disclosure Act – Health Service Circular 1999/198.* London, NHSE.

NHS Institute for Innovation and Improvement (NHS III) (2006) *NHS Leadership Qualities Framework.* Available from: www.institute.nhs.uk/index.php?option=com_joomcart&Itemid=194&main_page=document_product_info&products_id=246&Joomcartid=gu6si1nmtt4rlh5ubtif11j662 (accessed 11 July 2008).

NHS Institute for Innovation and Improvement (NHS III) (2007a) *Going Lean in the NHS.* Available from: www.institute.nhs.uk/option,com_joomcart/Itemid,26/main_page,document_product_ info/products_id,231.html (accessed 28 February 2008).

NHS Institute for Innovation and Improvement (NHS III) (2007b) *Releasing Time to Care: Productive Ward.* Warwick: Institute for Innovation and Improvement.

NHS Institute of Innovation and Improvement (NHS III) (2007c) *Transforming Good Ideas into Workable Solutions.* Available from: www.institute.nhs.uk/ (accessed 25 June 2007).

NHS Management Executive (1993) *A Vision for the Future.* London: DH.

Nicklin P (1995) 'Super supervision'. *Nursing Management,* 2 (5): 24–25.

Nursing and Midwifery Council (NMC) (2004a) *Standards of Proficiency for Pre-registration Nursing Education.* London: NMC.

Nursing and Midwifery Council (NMC) (2004b) *Midwives Rules and Standards.* London: NMC.

Nursing and Midwifery Council (NMC) (2004c) *Code of Professional Conduct.* London. NMC.

Nursing and Midwifery Council (NMC) (2006a) *A-Z Advice Sheet on Clinical Supervision.* Available from: www.nmc-uk.org (accessed 11 November 2007).

Nursing and Midwifery Council (NMC) (2006b) *The PREP Handbook.* Available from: www.nmc-uk.org (accessed 11 November 2007).

Nursing and Midwifery Council (NMC) (2006c) *Preceptorship – A-Z Advice Sheet.* Available from: www.nmc-uk.org (accessed 11 November 2007).

Nursing and Midwifery Council (NMC) (2007a) Statistical Analysis of the Register – 1 April 2005 to 31 March 2006. Available from: www.nmc-uk.org/aFrameDisplay.aspx?DocumentID=2593 (accessed 28 August 2007).

Nursing and Midwifery Council (NMC) (2007b) *NMC Advice for Delegation to Non-Regulated Healthcare Staff.* Available from: www.nmc-uk.org/aFrameDisplay.aspx? DocumentID=3076 (accessed 20 September 2007).

Nursing and Midwifery Council (NMC) (2008a) *The Code – Standards of Conduct, Performance and Ethics for Nurses and Midwives.* Available from: www.nmc-uk.org/ (accessed 9 May 2008).

Nursing and Midwifery Council (NMC) (2008b) *A Standard to Support Learning and Assessment in Practice.* London: NMC.

Odiorne S (1979) *MBO II:A System of Managerial Leadership for the 80s.* Belmont: Fearon Pitman Publishers.

Office of Public Sector Information (OPSI) (2005) *The Mental Capacity Act.* London: The Stationery Office.

Ogier, M E (1981) 'Ward sisters and their influence upon nurse learners'. *Nursing Times,* 2 April 1981, pp. 41–43.

Open University (2006) Course H812 [Postgraduate Certificate in Academic Practice] Glossary. Buckingham: Open University.

Orton, H (1981) 'Ward learning climate and student nurse response'. *Nursing Times,* 4 June 1981, pp. 65–68.

Orton H D, Prowse J and Millen C (1993) *Charting the Way to Excellence (Ward Learning Climate Project).* Sheffield: Sheffield Hallam University.

Palfreyman S, Tod A and Doyle J (2003) 'Comparing evidence-based practice of nurses and physiotherapists'. *British Journal of Nursing,* 12 (4): 246–253.

Parliamentary and Health Service Ombudsman (2007) *Annual Report 2005–06: Making a Difference*. London: The Stationery Office.

Pearson P, Procter S, Wilcockson J and Allgar V (2004) 'The process of hospital discharge for medical patients: a model'. *Journal of Advanced Nursing*, 46 (5): 496–505.

Pedler M, Burgoyne J and Boydell T (2007) *A Manager's Guide to Self-Development* (5th edn). London: McGraw-Hill Education.

Petersen A and Bunton R (eds) (1997) *Foucault, Health and Medicine*. New York: Routledge.

Proctor B (2001) 'Training for the supervision alliance attitude, skills and intention'. In Cutcliffe J, Butterworth T and Proctor B (eds) (2001) *Fundamental Themes in Clinical Supervision* (Chapter 3). London: Routledge.

Putnam R (1993) 'The prosperous community: social capital and public life'. *American Prospect*, 13 (Spring 1993): 35–42.

Rafferty A M, Clarke S P, Coles J, Ball J, James P, McKee M and Aiken L H (2007) 'Outcomes of variation in hospital nurse staffing in English hospitals: cross-sectional analysis of survey data and discharge records'. *International Journal of Nursing Studies*, 44 (2): 175–182.

Randle J, Stevenson K and Grayling I (2007) 'Reducing workplace bullying in healthcare organizations'. *Nursing Standard*, 21 (22): 49–56.

Resuscitation Council (2005) *A Systematic Approach to the Acutely Ill Patient*. Available from: www.resus.org.uk/ (accessed 11 November 2007).

Roberts K (2002) 'Exploring participation: older people on discharge from hospital'. *Journal of Advanced Nursing*, 40 (4): 413–420.

Robertson C and Finlay L (2007) 'Making a difference, teamwork and coping: the meaning of practice in acute physical settings'. *British Journal of Occupational Therapy*, 70 (2): 73–80.

Robinson G (1999) 'Leadership vs management'. *The British Journal of Administrative Management*, January/February 1999, pp. 20–21.

Rogers C and Freiberg H J (1994) *Freedom to Learn* (3rd edn). New Jersey: Pearson Education.

Rogers E and Shoemaker F (1971) *Communication Of Innovations: A Cross Cultural Report* (2nd edn). New York: The Free Press.

Rolfe G (1999) 'The pleasure of the bottomless: postmodernism, chaos and paradigm shift'. *Nurse Education Today*, 19 (8): 668–672.

Rotem A and Hart G (1995) 'The clinical learning environment: nurses' perceptions of professional development in clinical settings'. *Nurse Education Today*, 15 (1): 3–10.

Royal College of Nursing (RCN) (1996) *Clinical Effectiveness. A Royal College of Nursing Guide*. London: RCN.

Royal College of Nursing (RCN) (2005a) 'What is the clinical leadership programme?' *Clinical Leadership News (Newsletter)* Summer/Autumn 2004, p. 12. Available from: www.rcn.org.uk (accessed 11 November 2007).

Royal College of Nursing (RCN) (2005b) Maxi Nurses: Nurses Working in Advanced and Extended Roles Promoting and Developing Patient-centred Healthcare. London: RCN.

Royal College of Nursing (2005c) *Bullying and Harassment at Work*. London: RCN.

Royal College of Nursing (RCN) (2006a) *Practice Development*. Available from: www.rcn. org.uk (accessed 13 November 2006).

Royal College of Nursing (RCN) (2006b) *Setting Appropriate Ward Nurse Staffing Levels in NHS Acute Trusts*. London: RCN Policy Unit. Available from: www.rcn.org.uk/downloads/ policy/briefings/nurse_staffing_levels.pdf (accessed 13 November 2006).

Royal Pharmaceutical Society of Great Britain (RPSGB) (1997) *From Compliance to Concordance – Achieving Partnership in Medicine Taking*. London: RPSGB.

Saar S R and Trevizan M A (2007) 'Professional roles of a health team: a view of its components'. *Latin American Journal of Nursing*, 15 (1):106–112.

Sackett D L, Rosenburg W, Gray J M, Haynes R B and Richardson S W (1996) 'Evidence-based medicine: what it is and what it isn't'. *British Medical Journal*, 312 (7023): 71–72.

Sanderson H (2000) 'Information for health: information requirements for clinical governance'. *British Journal of Clinical Governance*, 5 (1): 52–57.

Scammell B (1990) *Communication Skills*. Basingstoke: McMillan.

Schon D (1995) *The Reflective Practitioner – How Professionals Think in Action.* Aldershot: Arena.

Scottish Executive Health Department (2003) *Effective Interventions Unit Integrated Care Pathways Guide 1: Definitions and Concepts.* Available from: www.scotland.gov.uk/Resource/Doc/47034/0013835.pdf (accessed 11 July 2007).

Scullion P (2002) 'Effective dissemination strategies'. *Nurse Researcher. Qualitative Approaches,* 10 (1): 65–67.

Shanley M J and Stevenson C (2006) 'Clinical supervision revisited'. *Journal of Nursing Management*, 14 (8): 586–592.

Shoup R (2000) *Take Control of Your Life*. London: McGraw-Hill.

Singleton J and McLaren S (1995) *Ethical Foundations of Healthcare – Responsibilities in Decision-making.* St Louis (Missouri): Mosby.

Sloan G and Watson H (2002) 'Clinical supervision models for nursing: structure, research and limitations'. *Nursing Standard*, 17 (4): 41–46.

Smith R (1992) 'Audit and Research'. *British Medical Journal*, 305 (6859): 905–906.

Snelgrove S and Hughes D (2002) 'Perceptions of teamwork in acute medical wards'. In Allen D and Hughes D (2002) *Nursing and the Division of Labour in Healthcare.* Basingstoke: Palgrave Macmillan.

Snow T (2006) 'Hewitt blames job cuts on trusts that employed "too many" staff'. *Nursing Standard*, 21 (12): 9.

Stewart R (1993) *The Reality of Organisations*. London: Macmillan Press.

Stewart R (1997) *The Reality of Management* (3rd edn). Oxford: Butterworth-Heinemann.

Stockwell F (1984) *The Unpopular Patient*. Beckenham: Croome Helm Ltd.

Stuart C C (2007) *Assessment, Supervision and Support in Clinical Practice* (2nd edn). Edinburgh: Churchill Livingstone.

Sullivan E J and Decker P J (2005) *Effective Leadership and Management in Nursing* (6th edn). London: Prentice Hall International.

Teamtechnology (2008) *Myers Briggs Personality Types*. Available from: www.teamtechnology.co.uk/myers-briggs/myers-briggs.htm (accessed 7 March 2008).

Thiroux J and Krasemann K (2007) *Ethics, Theory and Practice* (9th edn). New Jersey: Pearson and Prentice Hall.

Thompson C (1999) 'A conceptual treadmill: the need for "middle ground" in clinical decision making theory in nursing'. *Journal of Advanced Nursing*, 30 (5): 1222–1229.

Thompson C (2002) 'The value of research in clinical decision-making'. *Nursing Times*, 98 (42): 30–34.

Titchen A (2003) 'The Practice development Diamond'. In RCN (2003) *Annual International Nursing Research Conference Report.* London, RCN.

Tutton E and Seers K (2004) 'Comfort on a ward for older people'. *Journal of Advanced Nursing,* 46 (4): 380–389.

Tutton E M M (2005) 'Patient participation on a ward for frail older people'. *Journal of Advanced Nursing*, 50 (2): 43–152.

Vincent C A (2000) 'Reducing error in medicine'. Presentation at BMJ Conference, London. Cited in Department of Health (2000) *An Organisation with a Memory: Report of an Expert Group on Learning from Adverse Events in the NHS Chaired by the Chief Medical Officer.* London: The Stationery Office.

Wales S (2003) 'Integrated care pathways: what are they and how can they be used?' *Clinical Governance Bulletin*, 4 (2): 2–4.

Walsall Hospitals NHS Trust (2007) *Six C Model for a Good Patient Experience*. Walsall: Walsall Hospitals NHS Trust.

Waters K R and Luker K A (1996) 'Staff perspectives on the role of the nurse in rehabilitation wards for elderly people'. *Journal of Clinical Nursing*, 5 (2): 105–114.

Watkins K and Marsick V (1992) 'Building the learning organisation: a new role for human resource developers'. *Studies in Continuing Education*, 14 (2): 115–129.

Watson C M (1983) 'Leadership, management and the seven keys'. *Business Horizons*, March–April 1983, 8–13.

Webster J (2004) 'Person-centred assessment with older people'. *Nursing Older People*, 16 (3): 22–27.

Welsh M (2006) 'Engaging with peer-assessment in post-registration nurse education'. *Nurse Education in Practice*, 7 (2): 75–81.

West E, Barron D N, Dowsett J and Newton J N (1999) 'Hierarchies and cliques in the social networks of healthcare professionals: implications for the design of dissemination strategies'. *Social Science and Medicine*, 48 (56): 633–646.

Wheatley M (1999) 'Implementing clinical supervision'. *Nursing Management*, 6 (3): 28–32.

White R W and Lippitt R (1972) *Autocracy and Democracy – An Experimental Enquiry*. Connecticut: Greenwood Press.

World Health Organisation (2007) *News Release: WHO Collaborating Centre for Patient Safety Releases Nine Life-Saving Patient Safety Solutions*. Available from: www.jointcommissioninternational.org/24946/ (accessed 11 November 2007).

Wright, S (1989) *Changing Nursing Practice* London: Edward Arnold.

Wright S (1996) 'Unlock the leadership potential'. *Nursing Management*, 3 (2): 8–10.

Yoder-Wise P S (2003) *Leading and Managing in Nursing* (3rd edn). St Louis (Missouri): Mosby.

Yuen Loke A J T and Chow F L W (2007) 'Learning partnership – the experience of peer tutoring among nursing students: a qualitative study'. *International Journal of Nursing Studies*, 44 (2): 237–244.

Yukl G A (2002) *Leadership in Organizations*. Upper Saddle River: Prentice Hall.

Index